Endorsement

"Frank Harritt, a patient of mine since 2002, has an excellent working knowledge of diabetes treatment, including diet, exercise, and medication. Over the years he has demonstrated an outstanding level of diabetes control. I strongly recommend his book, *Diabetes Self-Defense*, to my own diabetic patients and to anyone with diabetes or pre-diabetes."

—Kevin Tong, MD, Board-Certified in Diabetes, Internal Medicine, Metabolism, and Endocrinology, Lakewood, CO

"When people receive the dreaded diagnosis of diabetes, so many think of it as a slow and painful death sentence. But author Frank Harritt says it doesn't have to be that way within the pages of his book, *Diabetes Self-Defense Weekly Journal and Reference Manual*. He educates you on what diabetes is and all the ramifications of having this disease, what you can do to stave off the ill effects of diabetes, what is optimally healthy to eat and drink when you are dealing with this diagnosis, how to prevent falling into some of the most common dietary and fitness traps, the importance of monitoring your key diabetes health markers, knowing what specific supplemental support you will need to implement, and why you should never stop learning about this disease that will be with you for the rest of your life. The key here is that your first defense in the battle over diabetes is *you* and you alone. Nobody is going to be able to control your diabetes better than the actions that you take. This book will help you get there."

—Jimmy Moore, *Livin' La Vida Low Carb Man*, Spartanburg, SC

"This is pretty cool."

—Rob Thompson, MD, Author, *The Sugar Blockers Diet*

"This book has been a great help to me in managing my diabetes; it's written in plain English so that anyone can understand."

—Carol Bradley, Columbia, SC

"This book has helped save my life."

—Gloria Bye, Arvada, CO

DIABETES
SELF-DEFENSE®

REVIEWED FOR MEDICAL ACCURACY BY JAY KRAKOVITZ, MD

YOUR ULTIMATE WEAPON IN THE WAR AGAINST
DIABETES!

FRANK HARRITT, MBA

DIABETES
SELF-DEFENSE®

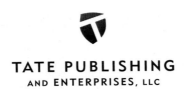

TATE PUBLISHING
AND ENTERPRISES, LLC

Published by Tate Publishing & Enterprises, LLC
127 E. Trade Center Terrace | Mustang, Oklahoma 73064 USA
1.888.361.9473 | www.tatepublishing.com

Tate Publishing is committed to excellence in the publishing industry. The company reflects the philosophy established by the founders, based on Psalm 68:11,
"The Lord gave the word and great was the company of those who published it."

Book design copyright © 2012 by Tate Publishing, LLC. All rights reserved.
Cover design by Matias Alasagas
Interior design by Jake Muelle

Published in the United States of America

ISBN: 978-1-62147-475-3
1. Health & Fitness / Diseases / Diabetes
2. Health & Fitness / Healthy Living
12.11.07

Dedication

I dedicate this book to God, the Great Physician, and all of the medical wonders He has wrought in the past and will provide in the future through his only Son, Jesus Christ. May all of God's children—of all ages, faiths, and races—who suffer from diabetes and pre-diabetes benefit in some way from the small part this book plays in the improvement of their diabetes knowledge and control. No matter how bad things may get for you with your diabetes, a key thought to keep in mind is that God will never leave or forsake you (New American Bible, Hebrews 13:5).

I sincerely wish to offer this book in loving memory of my late father and mother, William L. Harritt, MD, of Indianapolis, Indiana, who suffered from diabetes in later life, and Polly Moise Harritt of Sumter, South Carolina, who suffered from the effects of polio—infantile paralysis—almost her entire life. It was through their examples of perseverance and compassion as well as their emphasis on education that I developed a love for learning and a desire to help those who suffer. Finally, I would also like to dedicate this book to the memory of my late older brother, William L. Harritt, Jr., Esq., a rare attorney who practiced law with a genuine and deep compassion for those who suffer.

Acknowledgments

Diabetes Self-Defense® is protected under US Copyright Law, and copies, reproductions or other uses of this document are not permitted without the express written consent of the author.

The educational information contained within this website is not intended to be a substitute for professional medical advice. If you have diabetes or pre-diabetes, always consult your physician prior to making any changes in your diabetes management program.

While there are literally thousands of sources of information on diabetes for consumers and professionals, we selected the following list of experts on diabetes for use in creating and editing Diabetes Self-Defense®. Most of these expert sources are considered to be "top guns" in the field of diabetes care and yet also provide the average diabetic consumer with the best of conventional and alternative medicine for the management of diabetes that is supported by science.

The American Diabetes Association: it was through their series of professional publications and website (www.diabetes.org) that we were able to create our basic knowledge base.

The National Institute of Diabetes, Digestive and Kidney Disorders (NIDDK): a division of the National Institutes of Health (NIH). It was their excellent consumer modules and website at www.diabetes.niddk.nih.gov that provided us with substantial amounts of information.

The American Heart Association: especially in reference to their booklet, *Getting to the Heart of Diabetes*, a booklet on the increased risk of cardiovascular disease faced by people with diabetes, as well as from their very helpful website, www.heart.org/diabetes.

The Diabetes Research and Wellness Foundation® was founded to help and find the cure for diabetes and until that goal is achieved, to provide the care needed to combat the detrimental and life-threatening complications of this terrible disease. Their website is www.diabeteswellness.net.

The Diabetes Research Institute Foundation leads the world in cure-focused research and has made significant contributions to the field, which are used in diabetes centers around the world. The DRI translates promising findings from the lab to patients in the fastest, safest, and most efficient way possible. Their website is www.diabetesresearch.org.

The Johns Hopkins University School of Medicine: their superb series of medical white papers, including the one on Diabetes, by Simeon Margolis, MD, and Christopher Saudek, MD, was an essential resource. Johns Hopkins Hospital was recently ranked third for diabetes nationwide and their medical school first by US News And World Report. Their diabetes information website address is www.hopkinshospital.org/Diabetes/health_info.html.

The Mayo Clinic on Managing Diabetes: use of this book and the Mayo Clinic's website, www.mayoclinic.com, proved helpful in many areas, especially in the area of cholesterol and triglyceride management. The Mayo Clinic is consistently ranked at the top of America's most prestigious medical institutions in terms of diabetes care.

American Association of Clinical Endocrinologists (AACE) is a professional community of Clinical Endocrinologists that is committed to transforming the lives of patients by enabling one another to practice leading-edge, proactive, ethical, and cost-effective medicine. Their website is www.aace.com.

American Association of Diabetes Educators: The American Association of Diabetes Educators is a multidisciplinary professional membership organization of healthcare professionals dedicated to integrating successful self-management as a key outcome in the care of people with diabetes and related conditions. Their website is www.diabeteseducator.org.

The International Diabetes Federation (IDF) is the only global advocate for people with diabetes and their healthcare providers. Their mission is to promote diabetes care, prevention, and a cure worldwide. Their website is www.idf.org.

The website www.thepaleodiet.com: a consumer-friendly website that explains the basics of the Paleo Diet and how it can work for you from Loren Cordain, PhD. The theme of the website is "The Science of Healthy Eating," and it represents a viable diet for people with diabetes to consider.

The website www.diabetesmonitor.com: a consumer-friendly resource that literally surveys the web around the clock to provide the latest and greatest information on diabetes. Diabetes Monitor is run by William Quick, MD, and his wife, Stephanie Schwartz, RN, MPH, CDE.

The website www.bloodsugar101.com: an excellent web-based resource for people with diabetes by Jenny Ruhl, who has had diabetes herself since 1998. Jenny provides a wide range of informed information on diabetes, most of which you won't hear from traditional physicians.

The website www.medicalnewstoday.com: this health-based website provides up-to-date medical research and articles in a wide variety of fields, including diabetes.

7 Principles for Controlling Diabetes for Life, from the National Diabetes Education Program (NDEP), a joint program of the National Institutes of Health (NIH) and Centers for Disease Control and Prevention (CDC). Their website is www.ndep.nih.gov.

The website www.diabeteshealth.com: Published continuously for twenty years, *Diabetes Health* magazine provides objective, sometimes controversial, but always balanced articles about living with diabetes.

The website www.diabetes-normalsugars.com: the consumer-friendly diabetes site has been created by Richard Bernstein, MD, for the promotion of his low-carb programs, The Diabetes Solution and The Diabetes Diet. Check them out to see if they can work for you. Dr. Bernstein himself has had Type 1 diabetes for sixty-four years! You can find out more about his program at www.diabetes-book.com.

The website www.intelihealth.com: Aetna InteliHealth's mission is to empower people with trusted solutions for healthier lives. They accomplish this by providing credible information from the most trusted sources, including Harvard Medical School and Columbia University College of Dental Medicine. Established in 1996, Aetna InteliHealth has become one of the leading online health information companies in the world. Our health information includes health news and content as well as access to tools and risk assessments. Aetna InteliHealth is a subsidiary of Aetna and is funded by Aetna to the extent not funded by revenues from operations.

The website www.robkellermd.com is a site founded by the late Rob Keller, MD, one of America's foremost medical research experts on glutathione and the creator of the MaxGXL dietary supplement product.

The website www.lowglycemicload.com by Rob Thompson, MD, author of *The Low-Starch Diabetes Solution*, is an excellent resource for identifying the most common low glycemic load foods—the ones that are helpful in managing blood sugar levels.

Table of Contents

Part 5: "R" = Regular Medical Management

Part 6: "T" = Targeted Nutritional Support

Part 7: "S" = Study Diabetes!

Appendix

Diabetes Quotes of Note

Diabetes is a disease that, perhaps more than any other, depends much more on the patient than on the doctor.

—David Mendosa, *A Writer on the Web*, www.mendosa.com

Dramatic new evidence signals the unfolding of a diabetes epidemic in the United States. With obesity on the rise, we can expect the sharp increase in diabetes rates to continue to rise. Unless these trends are halted, the impact on our nation's health and medical care costs will be overwhelming.

—Jeffrey P. Koplan, MD, MPH
Director, Centers for Disease Control, 1998-2002

In total, only 7.3 percent of adults with diabetes in NHANES 1999-2000 attained recommended goals of A1c level less than 7 percent, blood pressure less than 130/80 mm Hg, and total cholesterol level less than 200 mg/dL.

—Sharon H. Saydah, PhD, Judith Fradkin, MD, and Catherine C. Cowie, PhD,
"Poor Control of Risk Factors for Vascular Disease Among Adults with Previously Diagnosed Diabetes,"
Journal of the American Medical Association, 2004; 291(3): 335-242.

The world is facing a growing diabetes epidemic of potentially devastating proportions. Its impact will be felt most severely in developing countries. The World Health Organization and the International Diabetes Federation are working together to support ongoing initiatives to prevent and manage diabetes and its complications, and to ensure the best quality of life possible for people with diabetes worldwide. Together we are helping to provide countries with the means to face the challenges that lie ahead. It is time for "Diabetes Action Now."

—Dr. Robert Beaglehole, World Health Organization, 2007
Professor Pierre Lefèbvre, International Diabetes Federation, 2007

Preface:
On Controlling Diabetes

Background and Overview

I am a board-certified internist who received his undergraduate and medical degree at the University of Pennsylvania. After completing an internal medicine residency at Lankenau Hospital in Philadelphia, I started a private practice in internal medicine. Having ultimately developed a three-person practice, I also concurrently served as Chairman of Medicine of Jeanes Hospital in Philadelphia. I was fortunate to be one of the first internists to participate in U.S. Healthcare's network in Philadelphia and was featured in one of the company's first television commercials.

I was soon thereafter recruited as a medical director after fourteen years of private practice in internal medicine. After Aetna merged with US Healthcare, I was named its interim Chief Medical Officer in 2000. In mid-2001, I left Aetna to pursue my interest in the growing Hospitalist movement and subsequently worked with two emerging companies. Most recently, I served as Anthem Blue Cross and Blue Shield Medical Director for Colorado and Nevada and Chief Medical Officer of Physician Health Partners.

I am presently serving on the Board of the Colorado Clinical Guidelines Collaborative, after having served three years as president. Today, I have also happily returned to the practice of Internal Medicine in Denver, Colorado, to more directly help my patients. As a person who himself has insulin-dependent diabetes, I personally understand the daily battles my patients face.

My Approach—Personalized Diabetes Care

In my medical practice, I see approximately thirty to forty diabetic patients per week. While it's true that we live today in an HMO world where many decisions are influenced by what insurance will or will not cover, I still maintain that the key to patient success is having personalized care in which the physician cares for his or her patients one at a time, one minute at a time, and this is especially critical for the patient with diabetes. Having been approached by the author of this book, I appreciated his wish to provide another way to reach the diabetic population with science-driven, yet consumer-friendly information.

I am also aware that he has had insulin-dependent diabetes for over twenty-four years—with no significant complications. The author, Frank Harritt, is the creator of Diabetes Self-Defense® and is a member of David Mendosa's diabetes support group in Boulder, Colorado, of which I have been a member for the last three years. In fact, it was in the diabetes support group that I, for the first time, actually heard from the patients themselves how they, in detail, were defending themselves against diabetes.

The Need in 2012...and Beyond

It's no secret that diabetes today has become a national epidemic, and groups from the American Association of Clinical Endocrinologists to WebMD have been citing the need for better solutions. While many of the cultural factors underlie the diabetes explosion—calorie-dense fast foods, a fast lifestyle, a less physically active population—it all adds up to a diabetes disaster, as Jeff Koplan, former director of the National Centers for Disease Control (CDC) saw years ago when he recognized the potential for diabetes to "overwhelm the US healthcare system."

Part of the Solution: Diabetes Self-Defense

Properly addressing the problem of diabetes (and its many complications) will require a convergence of public and private sector initiatives, with Diabetes Self-Defense® representing an excellent part of the solution. By empowering each diabetic patient to become the quarterback of their own diabetes healthcare team, with science-based education we can help them defend themselves against and minimize the short and long-term complications of diabetes. It is my hope that this book will provide a simple and easy-to-use guide for those suffering from diabetes and will give them the knowledge and confidence to manage their condition—using the most scientifically sound findings and approaches available today—in plain English.

Jay Krakovitz, MD

Introduction:
What is *Diabetes Self-Defense*®...Exactly?

Diabetes Self-Defense® is a practical tool for anyone concerned about defending themselves against the short and long-term complications of diabetes, whether the type of diabetes you are concerned about is Type 1 or Type 2. As the author of this book, I have been insulin-dependent for twenty-one years, having initially tried to manage my condition with diet, exercise, and oral medications. Today, with the help of Dr. Kevin Tong and my diabetes healthcare team in Denver, my diabetes is under good control, though I can never let my guard down, like you. But to win the twenty-four-seven War Against Diabetes, like any war, you have to fight on several *fronts*—weight, A1C blood sugar, blood pressure, and cholesterol. You must address the whole picture of diabetes, not just sugar (the "ABCs" of Diabetes—A = A1C blood sugar; B = Blood pressure; C = Cholesterol).

This combination book-journal is designed to help anyone with diabetes or pre-diabetes to get more education about their condition while simultaneously providing them with a tool for "one-stop-shopping" in terms of their diabetes management program: weekly education topics, weekly logbooks, medical checklists, medical records, and a diabetes glossary of commonly used terms. You may not need all of the charts and tracking forms, but they are there in case you do. Hopefully, this one journal will enable you to keep all of your diabetes medications and records in one place for easy and quick reference by your physician and diabetes healthcare team, helping them better assist you in your diabetes self-management program—and make you more successful. This is truly an "all-in-one" portable diabetes management tool.

Diabetes is a serious and deadly disease, but you can fight back. Having diabetes is like having ten diseases in one because it affects the blood and blood vessels, which touch every organ in the body. But with the help of tools like *Diabetes Self-Defense*®, you will be well-armed to fight back and win the war. Many myths about diabetes are still floating around, so the more educated you are with facts—not the myths—about diabetes, the better you will be able to defend yourself.

In today's HMO world, it is critical that the diabetes patient become *their own best doctor*. After all, in the world of diabetes care, the diabetes patient is the one who must monitor their blood sugar and blood pressure on a daily and weekly basis as well as administer their own therapy (nutrition, exercise) and their own medications (insulin shots, oral medications). That said, the recent ACCORD study, published in 2008, showed that *intensive control* of blood sugar, blood pressure, and cholesterol did not reduce diabetics' risk of cardiovascular events but did result in improvements with several microvascular complications (eyes, kidney, nerves). In other words, you need to develop the best medical targets for YOU with your doctor's help.

It no longer needs to be this way, where managing your blood sugar, blood pressure, and cholesterol are impossible to balance. By using this journal/log—much as you would any other health or fitness log—you can manage your diabetes on a daily basis while gaining a little bit of diabetes knowledge each week, to discuss with your doctor, your family, your friends, and other people with diabetes. And knowledge truly is power, power to help you control your diabetes instead of it controlling you. I am living proof that it can be done, because if someone like me can get good control of their diabetes, so can you.

The Purpose of This Book

This book is written as a tool for all people with diabetes or pre-diabetes to live the healthiest, happiest, and longest lives possible. For those with diabetes, it is designed to provide the proven yet simple "rules and tools" for effective diabetes management and control. For those with pre-diabetes, it provides the scientific knowledge—in plain English—that you need to help delay or entirely prevent the onset of full-blown diabetes. Pre-diabetes does not have to lead to full-blown diabetes, and full-blown diabetes does not have to mean severe complications. What happens to you short-term and longer-term is largely up to you and your diabetes team.

This book does not propose that it has all the answers to this complex disease, only that it offers hope to all those who struggle with it. Having diabetes no longer has to mean a shortened life of deprivation, denial, and depression, though it still can if it is left uncontrolled. Being a diabetic person doesn't mean you're an alien from the planet DiaBeta; to the contrary, people with diabetes can and should enjoy almost all foods and activities that their non-diabetic friends enjoy with few exceptions. There is no such thing as "diabetic diet" or a "wait, you can't eat that—you're diabetic!" What is good and healthy for you is also good for your non-diabetic friends. As a person with diabetes, I eat pretty much the same foods as everyone else with one little twist—I have to balance my food intake with my medications. If you need insulin, as I do, you also need to be especially careful about hypoglycemia or low blood sugar—meaning that you need to always be prepared by carrying glucose tablets or some form of fast-acting sugar with you wherever you go.

Make no mistake—*diabetes is a very serious disease*, and you must take it very seriously in all that you do, observing certain rules and guidelines. But the guidelines are not oppressive, nor are they necessarily difficult, despite the many myths that surround diabetes. It will take work on your part, but I am living proof it can be done, having had diabetes for over twenty-four years with no significant complications. And I am by far not the only nor the best example, for the Diabetes Prevention Program is scientific proof that a sound nutrition and exercise program can help prevent or alleviate the many complications of uncontrolled diabetes.

Prologue:
Using *Diabetes Self-Defense®* and Earning Your Black Belt!

Overview

Diabetes Self-Defense® is a tool for people with diabetes or pre-diabetes to defend themselves against the short and long-term complications of diabetes. Based on sound scientific information, this annual combination book/logbook provides weekly educational modules on the *right side* with a daily tracking form on the *left side* to record your blood sugar, blood pressure, exercise, and any illnesses. With blank forms and checklists in the *Appendix* for your medical records as well as your diabetes healthcare team and prescriptions, it is truly designed to be an all-in-one annual diabetes management and reference tool. It can help you and your doctor quickly and easily track your medical progress and make any adjustments that might be needed to help you gain better control of your diabetes—instead of it controlling you.

Recommended Method of Use

To help you get the most out of this book, the following process is recommended by the author:

1. Scan through the Table of Contents and overall journal to get the familiar with the weekly and daily layouts.
2. Read through the section up front—Diabetes 101—before you get officially started. It is designed to give you the big picture of diabetes before you get into specific aspects of the disease.
3. Flip through the medical charts in the back and fill them out with the names of the drugs you are taking, the names and numbers of your diabetes healthcare team, and the results of your last medical exam if you have them handy. These forms will be of great value to your physician and pharmacist in particular.
4. Begin reading the weekly topics and filling out your daily blood sugars, generally checking your sugar three to four times per day; this will give your physician a good idea of your blood sugar patterns and be able to make any medication adjustments, especially if your sugars are too high or too low. Try to fill out your blood pressure measurement once per week, but vary the time of day you check it. Most supermarkets and pharmacies today have free blood pressure monitors in their stores.
5. Skip around as needed. You may see a topic in the Table of Contents that is urgent for you, so read through that section as needed. While *Diabetes Self-Defense®* has been created to be used on a week-to-week basis as you go through the year, there's no reason you can't jump around as you need to.
6. The way to achieve Black Belt Status is to achieve *all* of your personal best A1C blood sugar, blood pressure, and LDL cholesterol goals at each medical exam, targets developed by you and your doctor for your unique situation. When all three are achieved at the same medical exam, you have qualified for a black belt degree. Over time, you can become a tenth degree, thirty-second degree, or fiftieth degree black belt—over a lifetime of exams. The more degrees you achieve, the better control you will have over your diabetes!

Best wishes as you now take better control of your diabetes through *Diabetes Self-Defense®* and work hard on getting your black belt in diabetes management.

Part 1:
Diabetes 101—The Big Picture of Diabetes

Diabetes 101 Summary

Before you dive into the War Against Diabetes, it's important to first get an overview or "the lay of the land." Diabetes is a disease that has been misunderstood and under-served for many years, and diabetes has gone from a *closet disease* to a full-blown epidemic in both America and the world in the last few decades. Before we can solve a problem, we need to understand the nature of the problem—who has it, why we have it, what caused it, and options for solving it. And while there is no cure yet for diabetes, there are many effective strategies to help us fight back.

Diabetes 101:
The Basics of Diabetes

What Are the Basic Facts about Diabetes?

There are a few basic facts that you need to know about diabetes, regardless of whether you are pre-diabetic, diabetic, or non-diabetic. Diabetes is a complex and serious disease, and today there is no known cure—only treatment. Diabetes appears in three basic types: (1) Type 1 (insulin-dependent); (2) Type 2 (non-insulin dependent); and (3) gestational, which occurs only during pregnancy. If left uncontrolled, diabetes can and does lead to long-term complications such as heart disease, stroke, blindness, amputations, kidney failure, and nerve disease. It is today the number three *contributor* to death in America according to the CDC, behind only heart disease and cancer.

However, modern scientific research has shown that many long-term complications can be minimized or prevented entirely through healthy lifestyle changes that include modest weight loss, regular exercise, and a healthy diet. Type 2 diabetes, which represents approximately 90 percent of all diabetes, largely results from obesity, poor diet/nutrition, and inadequate exercise over a long period of time. Sadly, more children today are being diagnosed with Type 2 diabetes than at any time in history. In America and worldwide, diabetes is now considered the number one heath issue and a genuine health epidemic.

Why Should I and My Children Be Concerned about Diabetes?

First of all, the life expectancy of a person with *uncontrolled diabetes* is approximately two-thirds that of a non-diabetic—which means a life expectancy of fifty-seven for the diabetic man and sixty-two for the diabetic woman. Aside from having a direct impact on the quality and length of your lives, there is another reason as cited by Dr. Jeffrey Koplan, Director of the CDC from 1998-2002: "Dramatic new evidence signals the unfolding of a diabetes epidemic in the United States. With obesity on the rise, we can expect the sharp rise in diabetes to continue. Unless these trends are halted, the impact on our nation's health and medical care costs will be overwhelming."

How Can I Gain Better Control of My Diabetes?

If your diabetes is currently not in good control, you need to see a doctor. A primary care doctor may treat you or refer you to a diabetes specialist known as an endocrinologist. With the assistance of your healthcare team, you need to follow the advice of the American Diabetes Association: "Know the ABCs of Diabetes" where the A stands for A1C (Blood Sugar); B stands for Blood Pressure, of vital concern to diabetics; and C stands for LDL Cholesterol, also a critical concern for diabetics. Modern medicine today acknowledges that diabetes must be treated with a multi-factorial approach—one that helps manage weight, blood sugar, blood pressure, and cholesterol simultaneously—and not with the old-fashioned approach of managing blood sugar alone. Blood sugar management is essential to successful diabetes care, but it is only one of several health measurements that needs close monitoring in people with diabetes.

Information Resources for Diabetes

1. The American Diabetes Association, "All About Diabetes" at http://www.diabetes.org/about-diabetes.jsp
2. The National Diabetes Information Clearinghouse, "Diabetes Overview" at http://www.diabetes.niddk.nih.gov/dm/pubs/overview/index.htmat
3. www.lifeclinic.com, "What is Diabetes—Diabetes Basics," at http://www.lifeclinic.com/focus/diabetes/about_it.asp

Diabetes 101:
The Overall Prevalence of Diabetes and Pre-Diabetes

What Is the Prevalence of Diabetes—in America and Worldwide?

According to the latest statistics from the American Diabetes Association, there are nearly twenty-six million Americans with diabetes or about 8 percent of America's population, and the vast majority are adults aged forty-five and older. In fact, in America, more than one out of every four adults sixty-five and older is diabetic. Worldwide, there are today 300 million people with diabetes, and that number is projected to grow to 500 million by 2030, according to the International Diabetes Federation (www.idf.org).

Diabetes is not isolated to one region of the world as it occurs in all races and socioeconomic groups, from the United States to Pakistan to England. In America alone in the past decade, diabetes has grown over 80 percent and today directly or indirectly affects nearly one in two adults overall. The picture is getting worse as diabetes has become a worldwide epidemic, and today there are 79 million pre-diabetics in America and 300 million worldwide. However, diabetes does strike at higher rates in Hispanic/Latino (10%), African-American (12%), and Native American adults (17%) in America. In 2011, there were slightly more American men (13 million) than women (12.6 million) with diabetes, but it is nearly a fifty-fifty split.

What Determines Whether One Is Pre-Diabetic or Diabetic?

While Type 1 diabetes can strike suddenly with the classic symptoms of increased thirst, unexplained weight loss, and increased urination, many people with Type 2 diabetes show no signs or symptoms. In fact, it is estimated that up to one third of people with diabetes do not even know they have it—nearly six million people in the United States alone. When symptoms for Type 2 diabetes do occur, they are just like Type 1 symptoms: increased thirst, unexplained weight loss, increased urination, especially at night, blurred vision, and sores that do not heal quickly. If you have any of these symptoms consistently and/or diabetes runs in your family, you need to be tested for diabetes at your doctor's office with a fasting glucose test—a test in which you do not eat for eight hours prior to visiting the doctor.

When your doctor tests your fasting blood sugar, if it's in the 70-100 mg/dL range, your test is normal. If the results are in the 100-125 mg/dL range, you are considered pre-diabetic and need to watch your situation carefully. If your fasting blood sugar is 126 mg/dL or higher, you are considered diabetic and need immediate treatment. However, remember that you cannot draw any conclusions from a single lab test; you need several lab tests with similar findings before you and your physician can confirm a diagnosis of diabetes. Additionally, certain drugs such as steroids and acute illness can also raise blood sugar.

How and When Should I Be Tested for Diabetes?

According to the US Surgeon General, anyone forty-five years or older should be getting tested every year for diabetes. If you are forty-five or older and overweight, it is recommended that you get tested immediately. If you are younger than forty-five but have several diabetes risk factors such as overweight, high blood pressure, Hispanic or African-American heritage, high cholesterol/triglycerides, and/or a family history of diabetes, you should consider testing as soon as possible. As you get older, your risk of getting Type 2 diabetes rises.

Information Resources for Diabetes Statistics

1. National Centers for Disease Control (CDC), National Diabetes Fact Sheet, at http://www.cdc.gov/diabetes/pubs/factsheet.htm.
2. The American Diabetes Association, National Diabetes Fact Sheet at http://www.diabetes.org/diabetes-statistics/national-diabetes-fact-sheet.jsp
3. National Diabetes Education Program, "*Overview of Diabetes in Children and Adolescents*" at http://www.ndep.nih.gov/diabetes/youth/youth_FS.htm

Diabetes 101:
The Types of Diabetes

What Does Scientific Research Reveal about The Different Types of Diabetes— Type 1, Type 2, and Gestational?

Type 1, Type 2, and gestational diabetes mellitus are the primary types of diabetes that affect 99 percent of all people with diabetes; the other 1 percent is represented by other forms.

Gestational diabetes develops only during pregnancy. Like Type 2 diabetes, it occurs more often in African Americans, American Indians, Hispanic Americans, and among women with a family history of diabetes. Women who have had gestational diabetes have a twenty to fifty percent chance of developing Type 2 diabetes within five to ten years.

Type 2 is the most common form of diabetes mellitus in the United States, affecting more than twenty million people. Both Type 1 and Type 2 diabetes cause high amounts of sugar (glucose) to circulate in the blood. Insulin produced by the pancreas is required to move sugar from the blood into the body's cells, where the sugar is used to create energy. People with Type 1 diabetes do not make enough insulin. People with Type 2 diabetes initially make plenty of insulin, but their cells are resistant to the action of insulin—the cells do not respond properly and high levels of sugar build up in their blood. Persistently high blood sugars make it hard for the body to fight infections and, over time, damage nerves and blood vessels, causing problems with the heart, brain, eyes, kidneys, feet, as well as other parts of the body.

Why Should I Be Concerned about Which Type of Diabetes I Have?

If you suspect you may have diabetes or pre-diabetes, the condition you experience just prior to acquiring full-blown diabetes, knowing which type you have will lead you to the best path of treatment and even potential reversal of the Type 2 if caught early enough; recent clinical trials such as the Diabetes Prevention Program (DPP) in 2002 have shown that losing weight, eating healthy, and getting adequate exercise can in fact minimize or prevent entirely the onset of diabetes. Nevertheless, the symptoms of Type 2 diabetes develop gradually, and some experts believe that pre-diabetes is often present for six to eight years before it turns into full-blown diabetes. Type 2 onset is not normally as sudden as in type 1 diabetes. Symptoms may include fatigue or nausea, frequent urination, unusual thirst, weight loss, blurred vision, frequent infections, and slow healing of wounds or sores. Some people have no symptoms whatsoever and discover their diabetes during a routine physical exam.

How Can I Prevent the Onset of Diabetes?

Per the positive results of the Diabetes Prevention Program, the best thing to do is to get your blood sugar (80-120 mg/dL), blood pressure (less than 130/80), and cholesterol (LDL cholesterol less than 100 mg/dL) into healthy ranges as soon as possible through losing excess weight, getting adequate exercise on a daily basis, and eating a low-fat, high-fiber diet rich in fruits and vegetables while carefully controlling calories.

The Types of Diabetes Information Resources

1. The National Institute for Diabetes and Digestive and Kidney Disorders at www.nih.niddk.org
2. The National Kidney Foundation or www.nkf.org
3. The American Diabetes Association (www.diabetes.org)

Diabetes 101:
Common Myths about Diabetes

What Are the Most Common Myths about Diabetes?

Some of the most common myths about diabetes are as follows:

Myth 1: You Can Catch Diabetes from Someone Else.

No. Although we don't know exactly why some people develop diabetes, we know diabetes is not contagious. It can't be caught like a cold or flu. There seems to be some genetic link in diabetes, particularly type 2 diabetes. Lifestyle factors also play a significant role.

Myth 2: People with Diabetes Can't Eat Sweets or Chocolate.

If eaten as part of a healthy meal plan, or combined with exercise, sweets and desserts can be eaten by people with diabetes. They are no more off limits to people with diabetes than they are to people without diabetes. Again, moderation and common sense are the keys.

Myth 3: Eating Too Much Sugar Causes Diabetes.

No. Diabetes is caused by a combination of both genetic and lifestyle factors. However, being overweight does increase your risk for developing Type 2 diabetes. If you have a history of diabetes in your family, eating a healthy meal plan and regular exercise are recommended to manage your weight and minimize your risk. Eating too many calories—too many carbs, fats, and proteins—all can contribute to the onset of diabetes when combined with low activity levels.

Myth 4: People with Diabetes Should Eat Special Diabetic Foods.

No. A healthy meal plan for people with diabetes is the same as that for everyone—low in fat (especially saturated and trans fat), moderate in salt and sugar, with meal plans based on lean meats, seafood, non-starchy vegetables, fruits, and nuts. "Diabetic" and "dietetic" versions of sugar-free foods offer no special benefit. They still raise blood glucose levels, are usually more expensive, and can also have a laxative effect if they contain sugar alcohols.

Myth 5: If You Have Diabetes, You Should Not Eat Starchy Foods, Such as Breads, Potatoes, and Pasta.

Starchy foods can be part of a healthy meal plan, but caution is needed; new evidence has revealed that low glycemic load diets that eliminate or minimize starchy foods are among the most effective for people with diabetes. The key is portions and number. For most people with diabetes, having three to four daily servings of low carbohydrate-containing foods is about right. Work with a nutritionist or dietitian to determine the portion size and number of servings for your unique needs.

Myth 6: People with Diabetes Are More Likely to Get Colds and Other Viral Illnesses.

Not necessarily, but it is true that people with diabetes, if their blood sugar is chronically high, may be more susceptible to certain bacterial or viral infections; the key is to keep your blood sugar as close to the normal range as possible. Also, people with diabetes are advised to get flu shots. This is because any infection interferes with your blood glucose management, putting you at risk of high blood glucose levels and, for those with Type 1 diabetes, an increased risk of ketoacidosis (lack of insulin in the blood).

Myth 7: Insulin Causes Weight Gain, and because Obesity Is Bad for You, Insulin Should Not Be Taken.

Both the UKPDS (United Kingdom Prospective Diabetes Study) and the DCCT (Diabetes Control and Complications Trial) have shown that the benefit of glucose management with insulin far outweighs the risk of weight gain.

Source: American Diabetes Association at www.diabetes.org

Diabetes 101:
The Obesity and Diabetes Crises

What Does Science Reveal about the Relationship between Obesity and Diabetes?

More than 85 percent of American adults with diabetes are overweight or obese, according to the U.S. Centers for Disease Control and Prevention. Obesity already affects 300 million people worldwide, and an estimated 750 million more are overweight.

According to Professor Pierre Lefebvre, President of the International Diabetes Federation, "The rise in Type 2 diabetes, is, in large part, due to weight gain." Not only does being overweight or obese significantly increase the risk of becoming diabetic, but once diagnosed, being overweight or obese makes the management of diabetes much more difficult due to the excess layers of fat and the higher levels of insulin resistance in the body. Health experts say that the twin global epidemics of obesity and diabetes are out of control and can reduce life expectancy in the future—despite the many recent advances in medical science. In the United States, the prevalence of excess weight and obesity among both adults and children has risen dramatically in the past two decades, but weight gain is not restricted to the United States. According to Dr. Lefebvre, some countries in the Middle East and Asia will also see a doubling of their overweight and obesity rates in the next thirty years.

Why Should I Worry about Obesity or Being Overweight?

The simple fact is that in America, nearly two out of three adults are overweight or obese, and 15 percent of adolescents ages twelve to nineteen are. Obesity and being overweight are not only risk factors for developing diabetes and/or increasing the risk of developing diabetic complications, but science has linked them to a higher incidence of heart disease and cancer as well. The greater the obesity, the greater the risk of major diseases. The estimated direct annual health cost attributed to obesity in the US is $147 billion, almost 10 percent of all medical spending. As you can see, obesity and diabetes pretty much work hand in hand.

How Can I Control Obesity or Being Overweight?

For people with diabetes, it is critical to lose a modest amount of whatever excess weight we have, even of just 5 to 7 percent. Science has shown that a small weight loss of only 5 to 7 percent can decrease or slow down the risk of becoming diabetic or developing complications such as cardiovascular disease, kidney disease, and some forms of cancer. Being diabetic, unfortunately, makes weight loss much more difficult than for a non-diabetic due to our *broken* metabolism and medications, especially if we are on insulin, which can promote weight gain. When it comes to achieving a healthy weight, whether you are diabetic or not, there are no quick fixes—no diet alone will get the job done.

Science has shown that 90 percent of people trying to lose weight permanently with diet alone will fail. So how do the 10 percent succeed? For people with diabetes, as with non-diabetics, the old equation of "calories in vs. calories out" determines whether or not weight is gained or lost. That said, of course, not all calories are equal, as noted in the recent best-seller by Gary Taubes, *Good Calories, Bad Calories*, a book that helps all of us better understand that the quality of our calories is also important.

Information Resources on Obesity and Diabetes

1. The International Diabetes Federation, "*Diabetes and The CVD Time Bomb*" at http://www.idf.org/node/1095
2. The American Diabetes Association, "*Weight Loss Matters*," at http://www.diabetes.org/weightloss-and-exercise/weightloss.jsp

Diabetes 101:
The Insulin Resistance Syndrome

What Is the Insulin Resistance Syndrome?

Metabolic syndrome, sometimes referred to as *Syndrome X*, is also called insulin resistance syndrome; it is widely considered today to be an underlying cause of Type 2 diabetes, which represents about 90 to 95 percent of all diabetics. Insulin resistance is a silent condition that significantly increases the risk of developing diabetes and heart disease, and it represents a diminished ability of your body's cells to adequately utilize insulin, the hormone that "opens the cell door" for blood sugar to enter as a source of energy. Because of this, the excess blood sugar stays in the bloodstream until it can be released from the body, normally through urine.

Medical researchers identify insulin resistance when any three of the following conditions exist: excess weight around the waist (40 inches for men, 35 inches for women); high triglyceride levels (150 mg/dL or higher); low levels of HDL or "good" cholesterol (below 40 mg/dL for men, below 50 for women); high blood pressure (130/85 mm Hg or higher); and high fasting blood sugar levels (100 mg/dL or higher). If you already have full-blown diabetes, you most likely already have three or more of these conditions that need immediate medical treatment.

Why Should I Be Concerned about Insulin Resistance Syndrome?

According to scientific studies, there are an estimated sixty to seventy-five million adults and children in the United States walking around with insulin resistance, putting them at high risk of developing diabetes or heart disease. After insulin resistance, pre-diabetes naturally follows, and then full-blown diabetes and/or heart disease. Studies show that most people with pre-diabetes go on to develop diabetes within ten years—unless they lose 5 to 7 percent of their excess body weight with healthy diet and exercise programs (see The Diabetes Prevention Program). People with pre-diabetes also have a higher risk of developing heart disease.

How and When Should I Get Tested for Insulin Resistance?

If you are overweight and forty-five years of age or older, you should ask your doctor about having a standard blood test that detects pre-diabetes and Type 2 diabetes as well as testing your blood pressure. If you are younger than forty-five and overweight, you may want a fasting blood sugar test to determine if you have pre-diabetes or diabetes. If your fasting blood sugar is over 100 mg/dL on more than one occasion, you are pre-diabetic; if it's over 125 mg/dL on more than one occasion, you are considered diabetic.

Diabetes normally takes five to eight years before it fully appears, but the sooner you learn about the presence of pre-diabetes or insulin resistance, the better your chances will be of avoiding it entirely or minimizing the impact of diabetes through a program of modest weight loss, a healthy diet, and moderate exercise or activity. The medication metformin has also been proven effective at delaying or minimizing the adult-onset of diabetes, though it is not as effective as weight loss, a healthy diet, and exercise.

Insulin Resistance and Diabetes Information Resources

1. The American Diabetes Association at http://www.diabetes.org/news-research/research/recent/ada-researchers-in-the-news/sugar-sweetened-beverages.html
2. The National Diabetes Information Clearinghouse, *Insulin Resistance and Pre-Diabetes*, at http://diabetes.niddk.nih.gov/dm/pubs/insulinresistance/

Diabetes 101:
Long-Term Diabetes Complications

What Does Science Reveal about the Long-Term Complications of Diabetes?

There are many serious, scientifically-proven long-term complications from diabetes: heart disease, stroke, blindness, kidney disease, nerve damage, amputations, periodontal disease, and a compromised immune system. In many ways, diabetes is the "king of diseases" as having diabetes is like having ten diseases in one. The reason is simple—diabetes as a metabolic disorder affects every major organ in the body and creates a massive level of biochemical chaos that threatens your health every day.

Why Should I Be Concerned about Long-Term Complications?

You should worry not only because uncontrolled diabetes can cut your life expectancy by as much as one-third, but also because you may be subject to a great deal of suffering and place a tremendous financial burden on your family along the way. The cold hard facts are that adults with diabetes compared with non-diabetics experience: (1) two to four times the risk of heart attack, and nearly two out of three people with diabetes die from heart disease; (2) two to four times the risk of stroke; (3) an extremely high probability of having high blood pressure and high cholesterol; (4) the leading cause of new cases of blindness among adults twenty to seventy-four years of age; (5) the leading cause of end-stage kidney disease; (6) a high probability of nerve damage, including to the heart; (7) the leading cause of non-traumatic lower-limb amputations, many of which are preventable with early detection; (8) a high probability of having periodontal (gum) disease; (9) a compromised immune system, making them more susceptible to bacterial infections of the skin, urinary tract and other organs; and (10) much higher than normal rates of depression.

How Can I Better Control My Diabetes?

Controlling diabetes today means a lot more than just controlling sugar. In the old days, doctors' primary treatment would be to tell their diabetic patients to "stop eating sugar." Yet today, diabetes has exploded—in a world full of sugar-substitutes. While managing blood sugar remains a critical part of every diabetes management plan, it is far from the only component. The American Diabetes Association (ADA) is promoting the *Know Your ABCs of Diabetes* campaign whereby the ABCs are: A = A1C blood sugar test, the test that measures your average blood sugar for two to three months and where your goal should be 7 percent or less; B = Blood Pressure, to keep it at 130/80 mm Hg or below; and C = Cholesterol, whereby you strive to keep your total cholesterol at 180 mg/dL or below with LDL cholesterol below 100 mg/dL. We also advocate adding "W" for weight control to the ADA prescription to create WABC-FM, like a radio station: Weight, A1C, Blood Pressure, and Cholesterol—For Me. In terms of weight management, it's good to strive for a BMI of twenty-five or less.

Information Resources on the Long-Term Complications of Diabetes

1. "A Look Back…and Forward," *Clinical Diabetes* 24:51-53, 2006, Jennifer Marks, MD, at http://clinical. diabetesjournals.org/cgi/content/full/24/2/51.
2. The National Institute for Diabetes and Digestive and Kidney Disorders or http://diabetes.niddk.nih. gov/complications/
3. The American Diabetes Association or Type 2 Diabetes Complications at http://www.diabetes. org/type-2-diabetes/complications.jspThe American Diabetes Association or Type 1 Diabetes Complications at http://www.diabetes.org/type-1-diabetes/complications.jsp

Diabetes 101:
Treatment of Long-Term Diabetes Complications

What Does Science Say about Treatment for the Long-Term Complications of Diabetes?

If diabetic complications arise over time, they need to be treated along with the diabetes itself as noted below:

Eye Disease of the Retina—Diabetic Retinopathy

One of the main treatments for diabetic retinopathy, which can cause blindness if left untreated, is laser treatment or laser photocoagulation, which can halt or stop the decline of vision in most patients.

Kidney Disease—Kidney Failure

There are four strategies for preventing or slowing the effects of kidney disease: (1) tight blood sugar control; (2) treating high blood pressure with diet and exercise; (3) restricting dietary protein; and (4) utilizing ACE inhibitors or high blood pressure drugs. Kidney dialysis is used for end-stage kidney failure—when kidney function falls to less than 10 percent of its normal function.

Nerve Disease—Diabetic Neuropathy

It is often difficult to treat the symptoms that result from diabetic neuropathy or diabetic nerve disease. Improved blood sugar control is the first step in treatment, often followed by different drug treatments for the different types of neuropathy.

Diabetic Foot Problems

Because people with diabetes often develop poor circulation in their extremities—like their fingers and toes—they are especially vulnerable to infections and gangrene in these areas. It is important to closely inspect your feet on a daily basis, especially if you get a cut. Your physician should examine your feet at least twice a year. Your physician will develop a treatment plan based on your unique situation.

Cardiovascular Disease

With few exceptions, preventive measures and treatment of cardiovascular disease are the same in people with diabetes as with non-diabetics, other than tight blood sugar control. Improved diet and exercise are usually the first line of treatment, followed by medications as needed, especially for high blood pressure and high cholesterol. Diabetes also produces changes in the blood that make it more prone to clotting, thus increasing the risk of heart attack or stroke; daily doses of aspirin from 81 mg to 325 mg are recommended to all people with diabetes. Angina—chest pain due to the reduction of blood flow to the heart—can be treated with drugs or surgery.

Source: www.healthmonitor.com

Diabetes 101:
Prevention of Diabetes and Complications

What Does Science Say about Preventing Diabetes and Its Long-Term Complications?

The Diabetes Prevention Program or DPP, with findings published in February, 2002, revealed that the onset and/or complications of Type 2 diabetes could be prevented entirely or minimized with either lifestyle changes or the use of an oral medication. In addition to achieving a healthy weight (Body Mass Index of twenty-five or less), the following steps have been shown to clinically reduce the risk of Type 1 and Type 2 diabetes complications:

- Blood Sugar Control: Research studies in the United States and abroad have found that improved glycemic control benefits people with either Type 1 or Type 2 diabetes. In general, for every 1 percentage point reduction in results of A1C blood tests, the risk of developing microvascular diabetic complications (eye, kidney, and nerve disease) is reduced by 40 percent.
- Blood Pressure Control: Blood pressure control can reduce cardiovascular disease (heart disease and stroke) by approximately 33 to 50 percent and can reduce microvascular disease (eye, kidney, and nerve disease) by approximately 33 percent. In general, for every ten millimeters of mercury (mm Hg) reduction in systolic blood pressure, the risk for any complication related to diabetes is reduced by 12 percent.
- Control of Blood Lipids: Improved control of cholesterol and lipids (for example, HDL, LDL, and triglycerides) can reduce cardiovascular complications by 20 to 50 percent.
- Preventive Care Practices for Eyes, Kidneys, and Feet: Detection and treatment of diabetic eye disease with laser therapy can reduce the development of severe vision loss by an estimated 50 to 60 percent.
- Comprehensive foot care programs can reduce amputation rates by 45 to 85 percent.
- Detection and treatment of early diabetic kidney disease can reduce the development of kidney failure by 30 to 70 percent.

Prevention of Diabetes Complications Information Resources

1. The National Institute of Diabetes and Digestive and Kidney Diseases or www.nih.niddk.org
2. The American Diabetes Association or www.diabetes.org

Diabetes 101:
The A1C Blood Sugar Test: Glycosylated Hemoglobin

Overview

Monitoring blood sugar levels and maintaining good blood sugar control are essential elements in the management of both Type 1 and Type 2 diabetes. Ask your healthcare provider to do a hemoglobin A1C test. This blood test shows the average amount of sugar in your blood over the past 2-3 months. Have this test done at least twice a year; some physicians like to have the test done every three months. Your healthcare provider uses this test plus your daily blood sugar records to tell if your blood sugar is under good control.

Aim for a score of less than 7 percent. If your A1C test result is 7 percent or less, then your blood sugar is where it needs to be and your diabetes treatment plan is working. A test result of 8 percent or higher is too high. At 8 percent or higher, you have a greater chance of having diabetes problems, like kidney damage, and you need a change in your diabetes plan. Your healthcare provider can help you decide which part of the plan needs changing. You may need to change your meal plan, your diabetes medicines, or your exercise plan.

What Is the Hemoglobin A1C...Exactly?

After a meal, glucose or blood sugar is absorbed from the intestine and circulates in the blood. Glucose is also made in the liver and released into the bloodstream in between meals. This glucose is normally used immediately for energy or it is stored for later use as fat or glycogen (sugar) in the liver. Some of the glucose attaches to hemoglobin, a protein found in red blood cells that carries oxygen throughout the body and gives blood its red color.

Blood sugar remains combined with hemoglobin for the life of the red blood cell—or about three months. The combination of blood sugar and hemoglobin is called glycosylated hemoglobin, or glycohemoglobin, or glycated hemoglobin. Its main component is HbA1c. When blood sugar levels on average are high, A1C increases. Because glycosylated hemoglobin stays in the blood for many weeks, measuring its levels gives a picture of average blood sugar control over the previous two to three months.

Only about half the people with diabetes have received the HbA1c test. If you have not yet received it, be sure to ask your doctor to schedule one for you. Historically, the only way to get an A1C test was to go to an authorized blood laboratory, but today many pharmacies carry home testing kits and many doctors have in-office labs. Consult with your healthcare provider to determine the best method for you.

Source: National Institute for Diabetes and Digestive and Kidney Diseases (NIDDK)

Diabetes 101:
The HEARTS Strategy for Fighting Diabetes

Overview

There are so many do's and don'ts associated with diabetes management that it can often be confusing. To help simply our strategies for fighting diabetes for life, *Diabetes Self-Defense* created the HEARTS strategy, a simple acronym that addresses the most serious health threat that people with diabetes face—cardiovascular disease (heart disease and stroke)—as well as the other multiple health threats (kidney disease, eye disease, nerve disease, amputations, etc.). Keeping our cardiovascular system healthy—managing our blood pressure and cholesterol—is just as important as keeping our blood sugar in a normal range. Recent studies have shown that most people with diabetes do not realize that having diabetes places them at a much greater risk of heart attack or stroke than the non-diabetic population.

The HEARTS Strategy: The Heart of Diabetes Self-Defense®

The basics of the HEARTS strategy, which serves as the premise for the design of *Diabetes Self-Defense*, are as follows:

- **H: Halt** or Minimize Vices. Too much smoking, alcohol, calories, caffeine, fried or fatty foods, cakes and cookies, and lack of exercise are bad news for people with diabetes or anyone else, but people with diabetes pay a much higher price than non-diabetics. While it's best to eliminate these vices completely, the next best thing is to minimize them whenever and however possible.

- **E: Eat and Drink** a Healthy Diet. Eating and drinking in a balanced, healthy way doesn't mean you need to be a health food fanatic; it simply means that, as a person with diabetes, it is essential to eat and drink mostly nutritious foods with proper portion control. It means you now have to pay careful attention to calories, carbohydrates, fat, and sodium content in what you eat and drink and most importantly eat a low-glycemic load diet.

- **A: Achieve** Common Sense Weight Loss and Fitness Goals. People with diabetes, in general, do not need to lose massive amounts of weight or run marathons to achieve good diabetes control. Research shows that moderate weight loss (5 percent to 7 percent) and moderate exercise (regular walking, gardening, biking) for 30 minutes at least every other day can help get and keep diabetes under good control. Consult with your healthcare provider on which programs are right—and realistic—for your lifestyle.

- **R: Regular** Medical Management. The ultimate success or failure of your *Diabetes Self-Defense* program can only be determined with regular medical management—led by you and supported by your diabetes healthcare team. Keeping accurate records of your weight, blood sugar, blood pressure, and cholesterol enables your doctor and healthcare team to help you gain maximum control over your diabetes. *Diabetes Self-Defense* is a tool to help you keep all of your annual medical records/changes in one simple book for quick, easy reference.

- **T: Targeted** Nutritional Support. Science from around the world has shown that certain supplements, like pycnogenol (pine bark), omega-3 fish oil, and antioxidants like Vitamin C can help fight heart disease and high blood pressure through their ability to help support normal levels of blood sugar, blood pressure, and cholesterol. Because people with diabetes have compromised immune systems, these extra weapons can help. One of the best researched lines of dietary supplements has been developed by a physician, Rob Keller, MD, and can be reviewed at our website, www.DiabetesSelfDefense.com.

- **S: Study** Diabetes! In order to manage diabetes effectively over the long haul, it's important to learn as much as you can about the disease. As in any other field, *knowledge truly is power*. We are fortunate to live in the information age, where diabetes knowledge is readily accessible over the internet; at the same time, always make sure that the diabetes information you receive is based on solid science and from a credible source.

Part 2:
"H" = Halt or Minimize Vices

H Section Summary

Many of the traditional vices in life—smoking, drinking, and drugs—can be especially dangerous for people with diabetes because of their compromised health condition. One additional vice that is especially noteworthy for the diabetic patient is overeating junk food—foods that contain extreme amounts of sodium, carbs, sugar, or saturated fat—or even too many sugar-free cakes and candies; sugar-free cookies, cakes and candies can contribute to weight gain. Blood sugar, blood pressure, and cholesterol are hard to control under the best of conditions, so the more you can do to eliminate or minimize the vices in your life, the more you will gain better control. In sum, beyond smoking or excessive drinking of alcohol, the greatest "vice" for people with diabetes is likely the overconsumption of refined carbohydrates, including but not limited to high-starch (bread, pasta, potatoes, cereals, corn, rice) and high-sugar (soda, fruit juice, cookies, cakes, doughnuts, pancakes/waffles) foods.

Reviewed by: **Jay Krakovitz, M.D.,** for:

DIABETES SELF-DEFENSE, LLC
6360 Quail Street, Denver, CO 80004
Cell: 303-931-9710; **Web:** www.DiabetesSelfDefense.com

Week Beginning: _____

Weekly Record

MON:	Time	Bld Sgr	Meals	Net Carbs(g)	2 Hrs Bld Sgr	Blood Press	Exercise/Min	Notes/Sickness
Breakfast								
Lunch								
Dinner								
Bedtime								

TUES:	Time	Bld Sgr	Meals	Net Carbs(g)	2 Hrs Bld Sgr	Blood Press	Exercise/Min	Notes/Sickness
Breakfast								
Lunch								
Dinner								
Bedtime								

WED:	Time	Bld Sgr	Meals	Net Carbs(g)	2 Hrs Bld Sgr	Blood Press	Exercise/Min	Notes/Sickness
Breakfast								
Lunch								
Dinner								
Bedtime								

THUR:	Time	Bld Sgr	Meals	Net Carbs(g)	2 Hrs Bld Sgr	Blood Press	Exercise/Min	Notes/Sickness
Breakfast								
Lunch								
Dinner								
Bedtime								

FRI:	Time	Bld Sgr	Meals	Net Carbs(g)	2 Hrs Bld Sgr	Blood Press	Exercise/Min	Notes/Sickness
Breakfast								
Lunch								
Dinner								
Bedtime								

SAT:	Time	Bld Sgr	Meals	Net Carbs(g)	2 Hrs Bld Sgr	Blood Press	Exercise/Min	Notes/Sickness
Breakfast								
Lunch								
Dinner								
Bedtime								

SUN:	Time	Bld Sgr	Meals	Net Carbs(g)	2 Hrs Bld Sgr	Blood Press	Exercise/Min	Notes/Sickness
Breakfast								
Lunch								
Dinner								
Bedtime								

Week 1:
Smoking and Diabetes

What Is the Scientific Relationship Between Smoking and Diabetes?

Tobacco has many bad health effects, particularly for people with diabetes. No matter how long you've smoked, your health will improve after you quit. Nicotine, the drug in tobacco, is one of the most addictive substances known. Besides the physical addiction, many smokers also become psychologically hooked on cigarettes. So kicking the habit is hard, but worth the work. There are many methods you can try to help you quit and stay away from smoking for good. If you smoke, ask your health care provider for help with quitting.

The best-known effect of smoking is that it causes cancer. Smoking can also aggravate many problems that people with diabetes already face, such as heart and blood vessel disease, as noted below:

1. Smoking cuts the amount of oxygen reaching tissues. The decrease in oxygen can lead to a heart attack, stroke, miscarriage, or stillbirth.
2. Smoking decreases HDL (good) cholesterol;
3. Smoking damages and constricts the blood vessels. This damage can worsen foot ulcers and lead to blood vessel disease and leg and foot infections.
4. Smokers with diabetes are more likely to get nerve damage and kidney disease.
5. Smokers get colds and respiratory infections easier.
6. Smoking increases your risk for limited joint mobility.
7. Smoking can cause cancer of the mouth, throat, lung, and bladder.
8. People with diabetes who smoke are three times as likely to die of cardiovascular disease as are other people with diabetes.
9. Smoking increases your blood pressure.
10. Smoking raises your blood sugar level, making it harder to control your diabetes.
11. Smoking can cause impotence.

What Can I Do to Cut Back or Quit Smoking Entirely?

There are many ways to quit: cold turkey or gradually, with a group or by yourself. Talk to your health care provider about your decision to quit. He or she can help you choose the best way for you. Remember, what works for one person may not work for another. Don't be discouraged if the first method you try fails. Another method may be the one you need to kick the habit for good.

One method that helps you quit gradually is nicotine replacement. When you wear a nicotine patch or chew nicotine gum, some of the nicotine enters your blood. The patch and gum let you taper off from the physical addiction slowly. They blunt your craving for cigarettes and reduce withdrawal symptoms. However, it is also well known that nicotine stimulates the heart and can raise blood pressure. If you have diabetes and are taking insulin, be sure to consult with your doctor prior to taking any nicotine product/patch.

Information Resources On Quitting Smoking

1. The American Diabetes Association on Smoking and Diabetes (http://www.diabetes.org/type-1-diabetes/smoking.jsp)
2. The National Diabetes Education Program at (www.ndep.nih.gov)

Reviewed by: **Jay Krakovitz, M.D.,** for:

DIABETES SELF-DEFENSE, LLC
6360 Quail Street, Denver, CO 80004
Cell: 303-931-9710; **Web:** www.DiabetesSelfDefense.com

Week Beginning: _____

Weekly Record

MON:	Time	Bld Sgr	Meals	Net Carbs(g)	2 Hrs Bld Sgr	Blood Press	Exercise/Min	Notes/Sickness
Breakfast								
Lunch								
Dinner								
Bedtime								

TUES:	Time	Bld Sgr	Meals	Net Carbs(g)	2 Hrs Bld Sgr	Blood Press	Exercise/Min	Notes/Sickness
Breakfast								
Lunch								
Dinner								
Bedtime								

WED:	Time	Bld Sgr	Meals	Net Carbs(g)	2 Hrs Bld Sgr	Blood Press	Exercise/Min	Notes/Sickness
Breakfast								
Lunch								
Dinner								
Bedtime								

THUR:	Time	Bld Sgr	Meals	Net Carbs(g)	2 Hrs Bld Sgr	Blood Press	Exercise/Min	Notes/Sickness
Breakfast								
Lunch								
Dinner								
Bedtime								

FRI:	Time	Bld Sgr	Meals	Net Carbs(g)	2 Hrs Bld Sgr	Blood Press	Exercise/Min	Notes/Sickness
Breakfast								
Lunch								
Dinner								
Bedtime								

SAT:	Time	Bld Sgr	Meals	Net Carbs(g)	2 Hrs Bld Sgr	Blood Press	Exercise/Min	Notes/Sickness
Breakfast								
Lunch								
Dinner								
Bedtime								

SUN:	Time	Bld Sgr	Meals	Net Carbs(g)	2 Hrs Bld Sgr	Blood Press	Exercise/Min	Notes/Sickness
Breakfast								
Lunch								
Dinner								
Bedtime								

Week 2:
Alcohol and Diabetes

What Is the Scientific Relationship Between Alcohol Consumption and Diabetes?

People with diabetes used to believe that alcohol was an off-limits item. However, modern research has shown that, if managed in the right way as part of an overall diabetes management plan, alcohol can be safely consumed in moderation by people with diabetes. A number of scientific studies have found an association between light to moderate alcohol amounts and decreased risk of Type 2 diabetes, coronary heart disease, and stroke in persons without diabetes. The greatest benefits of alcohol appear for people who engage in "light to moderate drinking." One drink of alcohol is commonly defined as 12 ounces of beer, 5 ounces of wine, or 1.5 ounces of distilled spirits (hard liquor). In other words, one should consume no more than one to two drinks per day. The key concept, though, between diabetes and alcohol is one of caution.

Studies suggest a "J" or "U" shaped curve: a small amount of alcohol per day is better than either no alcohol or a large amount of alcohol. The type of alcoholic drink doesn't seem to matter. Studies also report an increase in insulin sensitivity from moderate amounts of alcohol. Finally, studies indicate that light to moderate amounts of alcohol do not raise blood pressure, whereas chronic excessive amounts (greater than thirty to sixty g/day) do. The American Diabetes Association neither encourages nor discourages alcohol consumption for people with diabetes.

Should I Worry about Drinking Alcohol Occasionally?

Alcohol can potentially cause low or high blood sugars in people with diabetes. These effects are determined by the amount of alcohol acutely ingested, if consumed with or without food, and if use is chronic and excessive. In studies using moderate amounts of alcohol ingested with food in people with Type 1 or Type 2 diabetes, alcohol had no acute effect on blood glucose or insulin levels. Therefore, alcoholic beverages should be considered an addition to the regular food/meal plan for all people with diabetes, and no food should be omitted. If you take any drugs, even diabetes pills, ask your doctor about drinking safety.

If a patient has diabetes and is not already drinking alcohol routinely, he or she shouldn't start. If a patient has diabetes and already drinks a moderate amount of alcohol daily, he/she shouldn't escalate intake because high chronic alcohol intake (three or more drinks per day) can cause deterioration in long and short-term glucose metabolism. Heavy alcohol drinkers are strongly advised to reduce consumption.

If your blood sugar is not in good control, you should not be drinking any alcohol due to potential issues with blood sugar that can get too high or too low; for example, alcohol on an empty stomach can cause low blood glucose or hypoglycemia. Moreover, certain oral diabetes medications—sulfonylureas and meglitinides (Prandin) lower blood sugar by making more insulin. Your doctor can advise you on the safety of drinking when taking these and other diabetes medications, including metformin—one of the most widely prescribed diabetes medications.

Information Resources on Alcohol Consumption and Diabetes

1. Avogaro, A. *Diabetes Care*, June 6, 2004; vol 27: pp 1369-1374.
2. Wheeler, et al, *Alcohol Consumption and Type 2 Diabetes*, *DOC News*, October 1, 2004, Volume 1 Number 2 p. 7
3. The American Diabetes Association at http://www.diabetes.org/food-and-fitness/food/what-can-i-eat/alcohol.html

Week Beginning: _____

Weekly Record

MON:	Time	Bld Sgr	Meals	Net Carbs(g)	2 Hrs Bld Sgr	Blood Press	Exercise/Min	Notes/Sickness
Breakfast								
Lunch								
Dinner								
Bedtime								

TUES:	Time	Bld Sgr	Meals	Net Carbs(g)	2 Hrs Bld Sgr	Blood Press	Exercise/Min	Notes/Sickness
Breakfast								
Lunch								
Dinner								
Bedtime								

WED:	Time	Bld Sgr	Meals	Net Carbs(g)	2 Hrs Bld Sgr	Blood Press	Exercise/Min	Notes/Sickness
Breakfast								
Lunch								
Dinner								
Bedtime								

THUR:	Time	Bld Sgr	Meals	Net Carbs(g)	2 Hrs Bld Sgr	Blood Press	Exercise/Min	Notes/Sickness
Breakfast								
Lunch								
Dinner								
Bedtime								

FRI:	Time	Bld Sgr	Meals	Net Carbs(g)	2 Hrs Bld Sgr	Blood Press	Exercise/Min	Notes/Sickness
Breakfast								
Lunch								
Dinner								
Bedtime								

SAT:	Time	Bld Sgr	Meals	Net Carbs(g)	2 Hrs Bld Sgr	Blood Press	Exercise/Min	Notes/Sickness
Breakfast								
Lunch								
Dinner								
Bedtime								

SUN:	Time	Bld Sgr	Meals	Net Carbs(g)	2 Hrs Bld Sgr	Blood Press	Exercise/Min	Notes/Sickness
Breakfast								
Lunch								
Dinner								
Bedtime								

Week 3:
Caffeine and Diabetes

What Does Science Have to Say about Caffeine Consumption and Diabetes?

In research findings published in mid-2004 in *Diabetes Care* (July 26, 2004, vol. 34, No.6, pp.345-353), researchers at the Duke University Medical Center in North Carolina found that caffeine interferes with blood sugar control; they found a strong correlation between caffeine intake at mealtime and increased glucose and insulin levels among people with Type 2 diabetes. The findings are significant enough that the researchers recommend that people with diabetes consider reducing or eliminating caffeine from their diets.

One interesting side note from the study was that caffeine intake had little effect on glucose and insulin levels when the volunteers fasted but had a clear impact at mealtime.

Dr. James Lane, a psychiatry professor who led the study, observed this: "It appears that diabetics who consume caffeine are likely having a harder time regulating their insulin and glucose levels than those who don't" and that "it seems that caffeine, by further impairing the metabolism of meals, is something diabetics ought to consider avoiding. Some people already watch their diet and exercise regularly. Avoiding caffeine might be another way to better manage their disease. In fact, it's possible that staying away from caffeine could provide bigger benefits altogether." Dr. Lane and his colleagues studied fourteen habitual coffee drinkers with Type 2 diabetes.

However, for those who are not diabetic, a recent study by researchers at the Harvard School of Public Health and Brigham and Women's Hospital has found that participants who regularly drank coffee over the long-term significantly reduced the risk of onset of Type 2 diabetes, compared to non-coffee drinking participants. The findings appear in the January 6, 2004 issue of the *Annals of Internal Medicine.*

Should I Worry about My Caffeine Intake?

While researchers have differed in their caffeine conclusions over time, new evidence has strongly indicated that consumption of coffee and caffeine does not contribute to Cardiovascular Disease (CVD), finding neither caffeinated nor decaffeinated coffee associated with the risk of stroke—even for those drinking more than four cups of coffee a day. Moreover, a recent study in Finland even showed that people who drink coffee have a lower risk of developing diabetes (*Journal of the American Medical Association, 2002*). Besides caffeine, coffee contains magnesium, potassium, and antioxidants that may improve the body's response to insulin. Nevertheless, for people with diabetes, cutting back or quitting caffeine use appears to be a wise move, especially at mealtime. Caffeine-free drinks would be a better choice.

Caffeine and Diabetes Information Resources

1. Lane, et al, "Caffeine Impairs Glucose Metabolism in Type 2 Diabetes," *Diabetes Care* 27:2047-2048, 2004
2. Salazar-Marinez, et al, "Coffee Consumption and Risk of Type 2 Diabetes Mellitus," *Annals of Internal Medicine,* January 6, 2004, Volume 140, Issue 1: Pages 1-8.
3. DeNoon, D., "Caffeine Risks May Rattle Diabetic People," *WebMD.* Retrieved Jan. 28, 2008, from *http://diabetes.webmd.com/news/20080128/caffeine-risks-may-rattle-diabetics*

Week Beginning: _____

Weekly Record

MON:	Time	Bld Sgr	Meals	Net Carbs(g)	2 Hrs Bld Sgr	Blood Press	Exercise/Min	Notes/Sickness
Breakfast								
Lunch								
Dinner								
Bedtime								

TUES:	Time	Bld Sgr	Meals	Net Carbs(g)	2 Hrs Bld Sgr	Blood Press	Exercise/Min	Notes/Sickness
Breakfast								
Lunch								
Dinner								
Bedtime								

WED:	Time	Bld Sgr	Meals	Net Carbs(g)	2 Hrs Bld Sgr	Blood Press	Exercise/Min	Notes/Sickness
Breakfast								
Lunch								
Dinner								
Bedtime								

THUR:	Time	Bld Sgr	Meals	Net Carbs(g)	2 Hrs Bld Sgr	Blood Press	Exercise/Min	Notes/Sickness
Breakfast								
Lunch								
Dinner								
Bedtime								

FRI:	Time	Bld Sgr	Meals	Net Carbs(g)	2 Hrs Bld Sgr	Blood Press	Exercise/Min	Notes/Sickness
Breakfast								
Lunch								
Dinner								
Bedtime								

SAT:	Time	Bld Sgr	Meals	Net Carbs(g)	2 Hrs Bld Sgr	Blood Press	Exercise/Min	Notes/Sickness
Breakfast								
Lunch								
Dinner								
Bedtime								

SUN:	Time	Bld Sgr	Meals	Net Carbs(g)	2 Hrs Bld Sgr	Blood Press	Exercise/Min	Notes/Sickness
Breakfast								
Lunch								
Dinner								
Bedtime								

Week 4:
Sugar, Other Sweeteners, and Diabetes

What Does Science Have to Say about Sugar, Other Sweeteners, and Diabetes?

In 1994, the American Diabetes Association declared in their position paper that people with diabetes no longer needed to entirely avoid foods with refined sugar (sucrose); instead, sugar is allowed when consumed in moderation and as part of a well-balanced diabetes meal plan. The scientific evidence has shown that foods with refined sugar—like cookies or cakes—generally do not raise blood sugar any faster or higher than other types of carbohydrates like peas and beans. Sugars can be substituted for other carbohydrate food sources in the food/meal plan, or, if added, adequately covered with insulin or other glucose-lowering medication. Nevertheless, moderation is the key as foods like cookies and cakes are usually full of nutritionally empty calories.

You may have heard of the *Glycemic Index*, a measure of how fast or slow a particular food can raise blood sugar. However, the science is still mixed in regards to how eating a low glycemic diet can alleviate long-term complications, though it certainly couldn't hurt in the short-run. Remember, the old school of diabetes management recommended that diabetics strictly avoid sugar; today, we know that a more complete approach—controlling weight, blood sugar, blood pressure, and cholesterol—is a more sound method of diabetes management. A new book by Rob Thompson, MD, *The Sugar Blockers Diet*, shows how to use the *Glycemic Load* factor—which incorporates both the Glycemic Index and the amount of carbs per serving—along with other nutritional strategies to help support healthy blood sugar levels.

Why Should I Worry about Sugar, Other Sweeteners, and Diabetes?

All foods are eventually fully or partially converted to blood sugar or blood glucose as part of the metabolism process, so there is no need to worry about sugar alone, other than consuming refined sugar in moderation. In terms of sugar-substitutes and safety, the US Food and Drug Administration has thoroughly tested and approved five non-nutritive sweeteners for use in the US: 1) saccharin (like Sweet 'n Low®); 2) aspartame (like NutraSweet® or Equal®); 3) acesulfame potassium (or ace-K); 4) sucralose (like Splenda® or Sunett®); and 5) stevia (rebiana) as in the brands TruVia® and PureVia®.

A new form of sweetener used widely today is sugar alcohols, or polyols; these sweeteners include sorbitol, xylitol, maltitol, and mannitol and should generally be consumed in quantities of no more than three to six grams per serving. People with diabetes often mistakenly think that sugar free and no sugar added labels—which may be sweetened with sugar alcohols—will have no effect on their blood sugar, but they can. Not only that, when consumed in excess (nine grams or more per serving), sugar alcohols can cause severe stomach cramps and diarrhea due to their being difficult to absorb by the body. Even worse, many of the dessert products like *sugar-free* candies and chocolates are often loaded with deadly saturated fats and may be high in carbs. Make sure you review the entire label carefully prior to consuming such products, and do so only in small quantities. *Remember that sugar-free does not mean carbohydrate-free.*

How Can I Safely Incorporate Sugar Substitutes into My Diabetes Meal Plan?

Whether consuming sugar substitutes in foods or beverages, the key is *moderation*. In their latest recommendations, the American Diabetes Association has approved the consumption of all major sugar substitutes for people with diabetes other than saccharin for pregnant women and diet products like diet soda with phenylalanine for people with phenylketonuria.

Diabetes and Sugar Information Resources

1. The American Diabetes Association at http://www.diabetes.org/food-and-fitness/food/what-can-i-eat/artificial-sweeteners/sugar-free-claims.html

Reviewed by: **Jay Krakovitz, M.D.,** for:

DIABETES SELF-DEFENSE, LLC
6360 Quail Street, Denver, CO 80004
Cell: 303-931-9710; **Web:** www.DiabetesSelfDefense.com

Week Beginning: _____

Weekly Record

MON:	Time	Bld Sgr	Meals	Net Carbs(g)	2 Hrs Bld Sgr	Blood Press	Exercise/Min	Notes/Sickness
Breakfast								
Lunch								
Dinner								
Bedtime								

TUES:	Time	Bld Sgr	Meals	Net Carbs(g)	2 Hrs Bld Sgr	Blood Press	Exercise/Min	Notes/Sickness
Breakfast								
Lunch								
Dinner								
Bedtime								

WED:	Time	Bld Sgr	Meals	Net Carbs(g)	2 Hrs Bld Sgr	Blood Press	Exercise/Min	Notes/Sickness
Breakfast								
Lunch								
Dinner								
Bedtime								

THUR:	Time	Bld Sgr	Meals	Net Carbs(g)	2 Hrs Bld Sgr	Blood Press	Exercise/Min	Notes/Sickness
Breakfast								
Lunch								
Dinner								
Bedtime								

FRI:	Time	Bld Sgr	Meals	Net Carbs(g)	2 Hrs Bld Sgr	Blood Press	Exercise/Min	Notes/Sickness
Breakfast								
Lunch								
Dinner								
Bedtime								

SAT:	Time	Bld Sgr	Meals	Net Carbs(g)	2 Hrs Bld Sgr	Blood Press	Exercise/Min	Notes/Sickness
Breakfast								
Lunch								
Dinner								
Bedtime								

SUN:	Time	Bld Sgr	Meals	Net Carbs(g)	2 Hrs Bld Sgr	Blood Press	Exercise/Min	Notes/Sickness
Breakfast								
Lunch								
Dinner								
Bedtime								

Week 5:
Fast Foods, Special Occasions, and Diabetes

What Does Science Say about Fast Foods, Special Occasions, and Diabetes?

While the explosion of diabetes in the past decade in America cannot be solely linked to the fast food mega-meals (*Super-Size Me*), there is evidence that links the western-style diet, including fast food—to Type 2 diabetes incidence. In the study, the western diet is described as embracing red meat, desserts, high-fat dairy products, and processed foods—a definition that includes the classic junk foods like hamburgers, doughnuts, French fries, fried chicken, pies, cakes, ice cream, and potato chips/snack foods—many high-starch and high-sugar foods; coincidentally, these are the types of foods most often consumed on special occasions and major holidays.

The implications of the study were that to decrease their chances of getting Type 2 diabetes, people should increase their intake of vegetables, fruits, fish, and poultry, and limit intake of red meat, processed meat, high-fat dairy foods, refined grains, and sweets. Plain and simple, fast foods and holiday foods tend to be high in sugar, starch, saturated fat, and sodium—items that all diabetics need to minimize in their meal plans.

Why Should I Be Concerned about Fast Foods and Special Occasion Foods?

Make no mistake—the hard facts show us that regular consumption of the "Western-style diet" puts us at greater risk of developing diabetes as well as contributing to long-term complications if we already have it. And while all of the scientific data is critical, it must also be kept in a common-sense perspective. For special occasions such as birthdays and major holidays—events that may occur on one or two times per month on average—having a small serving (3 oz.) of a fast food or holiday food will not ruin your diabetes management program, but the portion or serving size must be kept small and managed within your overall meal plan. In his book, *The Low-Starch Diabetes Solution*, Dr. Rob Thompson, himself a diabetic, suggests that a small square of dark chocolate at the end of a meal may even have some health benefits.

If you are going to have a piece of cake or pie over the holidays or at a company party, you simply need to plan ahead with your meal plan and medications. Having diabetes no longer means that you can *never* have fast foods or holiday foods, but it does mean you have to do so with greater planning than ever before. And rather than eating a treat as a single item, make sure you combine it into a full meal occasion whenever possible. Additionally, on those days where you do include special foods or treats, try to get some additional physical exercise as well.

Fast Foods and Diabetes Information Resources

1. van Dam, et al, "Dietary Patterns and Risk for Type 2 Diabetes Mellitus in U.S. Men," February 5, 2002, *Annals of Internal Medicine*, Vol. 136, Issue 3, pp.201-209)M. A. Pereira, et al, "Fast-food habits, weight gain, and insulin resistance (the CARDIA study): 15-year prospective analysis." *Lancet* 2005; 365: 36-42.
2. www.diabetes-and-diet.com (especially good for kids with diabetes)

Part 3:
"E" = Eating and Drinking a Healthy Diet

E Section Summary

In the War Against Diabetes, there is no weapon more powerful than a healthy, well-balanced diet. Medications can help, and exercise can be a valuable tool, but nothing will help you gain better control of your weight, blood sugar, blood pressure, and cholesterol than your diet. No matter where you are in your personal diabetes management program, improving the foods and beverages that you consume will go a long way toward helping you gain better control. While there is no "one diet" for people with diabetes, it has now been acknowledged—even by the American Diabetes Association—that a low-carb diet can help produce weight loss.

Other studies have shown that a low-carb diet can also help improve weight, blood sugar, blood pressure, and cholesterol levels in people with diabetes. Our research has shown that one of the best overall diets—for people with diabetes/pre-diabetes or any compromised health condition such as heart disease, high blood pressure, cancer, or obesity—is the scientifically supported, low-carb *Paleo Diet* from Loren Cordain, PhD, at Colorado State University, an approach that leverages the proven health-promoting principles derived from the diet and exercise habits of our Paleolithic (Old Stone Age) ancestors. Another very sound dietary approach for diabetes management is from Rob Thompson, MD, in his book *The Low-Starch Diabetes Solution*; Dr. Thompson is himself a diabetic, so he knows personally about the battles faced by his diabetic patients.

Week Beginning: _____

Weekly Record

MON:	Time	Bld Sgr	Meals	Net Carbs(g)	2 Hrs Bld Sgr	Blood Press	Exercise/Min	Notes/Sickness
Breakfast								
Lunch								
Dinner								
Bedtime								

TUES:	Time	Bld Sgr	Meals	Net Carbs(g)	2 Hrs Bld Sgr	Blood Press	Exercise/Min	Notes/Sickness
Breakfast								
Lunch								
Dinner								
Bedtime								

WED:	Time	Bld Sgr	Meals	Net Carbs(g)	2 Hrs Bld Sgr	Blood Press	Exercise/Min	Notes/Sickness
Breakfast								
Lunch								
Dinner								
Bedtime								

THUR:	Time	Bld Sgr	Meals	Net Carbs(g)	2 Hrs Bld Sgr	Blood Press	Exercise/Min	Notes/Sickness
Breakfast								
Lunch								
Dinner								
Bedtime								

FRI:	Time	Bld Sgr	Meals	Net Carbs(g)	2 Hrs Bld Sgr	Blood Press	Exercise/Min	Notes/Sickness
Breakfast								
Lunch								
Dinner								
Bedtime								

SAT:	Time	Bld Sgr	Meals	Net Carbs(g)	2 Hrs Bld Sgr	Blood Press	Exercise/Min	Notes/Sickness
Breakfast								
Lunch								
Dinner								
Bedtime								

SUN:	Time	Bld Sgr	Meals	Net Carbs(g)	2 Hrs Bld Sgr	Blood Press	Exercise/Min	Notes/Sickness
Breakfast								
Lunch								
Dinner								
Bedtime								

Week 6:
Evidence-Based Nutrition Principles

What Does Science Say about Nutrition and Diabetes?

Medical nutrition therapy (MNT) is an integral component of diabetes management and of diabetes self-management education. Yet many misconceptions exist concerning nutrition and diabetes. Moreover, in clinical practice, nutrition recommendations that have little or no supporting evidence have been and are still being given to persons with diabetes. Accordingly, a position statement has been developed by the American Diabetes Association that provides evidence-based principles and recommendations for diabetes medical nutrition therapy. The rationale for this position statement is discussed in the American Diabetes Association technical review "Evidence-Based Nutrition Principles and Recommendations for the Treatment and Prevention of Diabetes and Related Complications," which discusses in detail the published research for each principle and recommendation.

Why Should I Be Concerned about Nutrition?

While good nutrition is clearly not an issue for diabetics only, if you have diabetes (or impaired glucose tolerance), your blood sugar can get dangerously high or low. If your blood sugar goes too high or too low, you can get very sick. Your blood sugar gets too high or too low if you don't take the right amount of diabetes medicine in relation to the amount of food you are eating or beverage you are drinking, such as a meal replacement shake, glass of milk, or mixed drink. If your blood sugar stays high too much of the time, you can get heart, eye, foot, kidney, and other problems. You can also have serious problems if your blood sugar gets too low (hypoglycemia) too often. Keeping your blood sugar as close to normal as possible (80-120 mg/dL) will prevent or slow down diabetes problems.

How Can I Develop a Good Nutritional Plan for My Unique Needs?

Because of the complexity of nutrition issues, it is recommended that a registered dietitian or Certified Diabetes Educator (CDE, knowledgeable and skilled in implementing nutrition therapy into diabetes management and education) be the team member providing medical nutrition therapy. However, it is essential that all diabetes team members be knowledgeable about nutrition therapy and supportive of the person with diabetes who needs to make lifestyle changes. As a general rule, you should try to consume a diet that is high in good fats, high in fiber, rich in vitamins, minerals, and phytonutrients, and low in carbohydrates, especially those that are refined. Finally, as important as nutritional wisdom is for effective blood sugar management, never forget that exercise/activity, beverages, and medications also play a vital role when it comes to achieving and maintaining effective blood sugar, blood pressure, and cholesterol control.

Nutrition and Diabetes Information Resources

1. The American Diabetes Association Position Statement: "Evidence-Based Nutrition Principles and Recommendations for the Treatment and Prevention of Diabetes and Related Complications," *Diabetes Care* 25:202-212, 2002
2. Cordain, Loren, Ph.D., *The Paleo Diet*, ©2002, John Wiley and Sons, or www.thepaleodiet.com.
3. Thompson, Rob, MD, *The Low-Starch Diabetes Solution*, ©2010, McGraw-Hill Books, or www.lowglycemicload.com

Reviewed by: **Jay Krakovitz, M.D.,** for:

DIABETES SELF-DEFENSE, LLC
6360 Quail Street, Denver, CO 80004
Cell: 303-931-9710; **Web:** www.DiabetesSelfDefense.com

Week Beginning: _____

Weekly Record

MON:	Time	Bld Sgr	Meals	Net Carbs(g)	2 Hrs Bld Sgr	Blood Press	Exercise/Min	Notes/Sickness
Breakfast								
Lunch								
Dinner								
Bedtime								

TUES:	Time	Bld Sgr	Meals	Net Carbs(g)	2 Hrs Bld Sgr	Blood Press	Exercise/Min	Notes/Sickness
Breakfast								
Lunch								
Dinner								
Bedtime								

WED:	Time	Bld Sgr	Meals	Net Carbs(g)	2 Hrs Bld Sgr	Blood Press	Exercise/Min	Notes/Sickness
Breakfast								
Lunch								
Dinner								
Bedtime								

THUR:	Time	Bld Sgr	Meals	Net Carbs(g)	2 Hrs Bld Sgr	Blood Press	Exercise/Min	Notes/Sickness
Breakfast								
Lunch								
Dinner								
Bedtime								

FRI:	Time	Bld Sgr	Meals	Net Carbs(g)	2 Hrs Bld Sgr	Blood Press	Exercise/Min	Notes/Sickness
Breakfast								
Lunch								
Dinner								
Bedtime								

SAT:	Time	Bld Sgr	Meals	Net Carbs(g)	2 Hrs Bld Sgr	Blood Press	Exercise/Min	Notes/Sickness
Breakfast								
Lunch								
Dinner								
Bedtime								

SUN:	Time	Bld Sgr	Meals	Net Carbs(g)	2 Hrs Bld Sgr	Blood Press	Exercise/Min	Notes/Sickness
Breakfast								
Lunch								
Dinner								
Bedtime								

Week 7:
Healthy Food Preparation for Diabetes

What Are the Best Ways for Diabetics to Enjoy Tasty and Healthy Meals?

A few simple meal planning and preparation tips will help you to produce healthy, delicious food that your family will love. Five key steps highlighted by the Canadian Diabetes Association are as follows:

1. Take a few minutes each week to plan your menus. This will allow you the time to schedule a quick and easy meal for the times when you and your children have extracurricular activities, from soccer matches to parent-teacher meetings. As well, you will be able to try a new recipe or ensure that a favorite is served more often.

2. Choose seasonal produce and pick the brightest colors that you can. Buying fruits and vegetables in season lets you enjoy peak flavor at modest cost. Buy asparagus in the spring, peaches in the late summer, and apples in the fall. When the price of fresh produce is high, frozen fruit and vegetables are usually an economical choice. Canned fruit and vegetables are another alternative, but be aware of the sugary syrups and higher salt content. Fruits and vegetables provide lots of vitamins and minerals to keep you healthy at a very modest calorie cost. In general, the darker the color, the higher the nutrients (think bright red peppers, or dark green broccoli).

3. Use cooking methods that do not add extra fat to the dish. Steamed vegetables are especially flavorful when herbs are added to the steaming liquid. Broiled or grilled meats are lower in fat and develop a rich golden color that adds visual and taste appeal. Baking, especially in a pan with a rack is another low fat cooking method. The microwave allows you to prepare food quickly without added fat. Barbecuing is another lower calorie cooking method.

4. Reduce or eliminate high fat ingredients from your favorite recipes. Using a non-stick pan means that you can sauté without added fat. Adding tofu, bulgur, or brown rice to casseroles means that you can cut down on the amount of meat that you are using. Using smaller amounts of stronger cheeses decreases the amount of milder cheese needed without sacrificing the flavor. Chilling a soup or stew will allow the fat to rise to the top and congeal for easy removal.

5. Learn to use spices and herbs to kick up the flavor. Parsley, sage, rosemary, and thyme are classic herbs that you will savor. Cinnamon, cloves, and nutmeg will add a new taste to traditional dishes. Many cookbooks offer advice on using spices and herbs and many recipes on the internet will introduce new tastes.

Healthy Diabetic Food Preparation Information Sources

1. The Canadian Diabetes Association at www.diabetes.ca
2. The American Diabetes Association at www.diabetes.org
3. Diabetic Gourmet Magazine (www.diabeticgourmet.com)

Reviewed by: **Jay Krakovitz, M.D.,** for:

DIABETES SELF-DEFENSE, LLC
6360 Quail Street, Denver, CO 80004
Cell: 303-931-9710; **Web:** www.DiabetesSelfDefense.com

Week Beginning: _____

Weekly Record

MON:	Time	Bld Sgr	Meals	Net Carbs(g)	2 Hrs Bld Sgr	Blood Press	Exercise/Min	Notes/Sickness
Breakfast								
Lunch								
Dinner								
Bedtime								

TUES:	Time	Bld Sgr	Meals	Net Carbs(g)	2 Hrs Bld Sgr	Blood Press	Exercise/Min	Notes/Sickness
Breakfast								
Lunch								
Dinner								
Bedtime								

WED:	Time	Bld Sgr	Meals	Net Carbs(g)	2 Hrs Bld Sgr	Blood Press	Exercise/Min	Notes/Sickness
Breakfast								
Lunch								
Dinner								
Bedtime								

THUR:	Time	Bld Sgr	Meals	Net Carbs(g)	2 Hrs Bld Sgr	Blood Press	Exercise/Min	Notes/Sickness
Breakfast								
Lunch								
Dinner								
Bedtime								

FRI:	Time	Bld Sgr	Meals	Net Carbs(g)	2 Hrs Bld Sgr	Blood Press	Exercise/Min	Notes/Sickness
Breakfast								
Lunch								
Dinner								
Bedtime								

SAT:	Time	Bld Sgr	Meals	Net Carbs(g)	2 Hrs Bld Sgr	Blood Press	Exercise/Min	Notes/Sickness
Breakfast								
Lunch								
Dinner								
Bedtime								

SUN:	Time	Bld Sgr	Meals	Net Carbs(g)	2 Hrs Bld Sgr	Blood Press	Exercise/Min	Notes/Sickness
Breakfast								
Lunch								
Dinner								
Bedtime								

Week 8:
Carbohydrate and Fiber Recommendations for Diabetes

What Does Science Say about Carbohydrate/Fiber Consumption and Diabetes?

Based on the scientific analyses of many clinical studies with diabetics, Dr. James W. Anderson and his associates at the University of Kentucky College of Medicine, Department of Internal Medicine, recommend that the diabetic individual should be encouraged to achieve and maintain a desirable body weight (BMI of less than twenty-five) and that the diet should provide these percentages of nutrients: carbohydrate, greater than or equal to 55 percent; protein, 12 to 16 percent; fat, less than 30 percent; and monounsaturated fat, 12 to 15 percent. The diet should provide twenty-five to fifty grams/day of dietary fiber (15-25 grams/1000 kcal).

However, there are also several alternative diet plans to consider, such as *Dr. Bernstein's Diabetes Solution* by Dr. Richard Bernstein, *The Paleo Diet* by Dr. Loren Cordain, and *The Low-Starch Diabetes Solution* by Rob Thompson, MD, all of which are viable options for a person with diabetes to consider. These diets advocate the importance of a low-carb or very-low carb diet for people with diabetes and offer strong levels of scientific support for their positions.

Why Should I Be Concerned about Carbohydrate and Fiber Consumption?

For diabetic subjects, low-to-moderate carbohydrate, high-fiber diets compared to high carbohydrate, low-fiber diets are associated with *significantly lower values* for: post-meal blood glucose, total and low-density lipoprotein cholesterol (LDL or *bad* cholesterol), high-density lipoprotein cholesterol (HDL or "good" cholesterol), and triglycerides. Low-to-moderate carbohydrate, high-fiber diets compared to high carbohydrate, low-fiber diets are associated with lower values for: fasting, post-meal and average plasma glucose; hemoglobin A1C; total, LDL-cholesterol, HDL-cholesterol; and triglycerides.

While high-fat, low-carb diets like Atkins may promote a short-term weight loss, the potential hazards for worsening risk for progression of atherosclerosis or coronary heart disease (CHD) override the short-term benefits. Individuals derive the greatest health benefits from diets low in saturated fat and high in fiber; these increase sensitivity to insulin and lower risk for CHD. In fact, at the end of 2007 the American Diabetes Association officially endorsed either a low-carb or low-fat dietary approach to help lose weight on a short-term basis, which is the first time the organization has endorsed the low-carb approach in any form (www.diabetes.org).

How Can I Get Adequate Amounts of Carbohydrates and Fiber in My Diet?

As part of managing your diabetes, make sure you are eating a balanced and varied diet—based on your unique caloric requirements—that includes significant amounts of fruits and vegetables as the foundation; your doctor and dietitian can work with you to develop a specific meal plan that best fits your lifestyle. *The Paleo Diet* by Dr. Loren Cordain is considered to be one of the more effective—though certainly not the only—low-carb approaches for the management of diabetes as it emphasizes the careful integration of lean meats, seafood, fruits, non-starchy vegetables, and nuts—the same basic diet eaten by our Stone Age ancestors. Following this diet/lifestyle will allow you to eat a wide variety of delicious, healthy foods while ensuring that your diet is rich in vitamins, minerals, and fiber, and an additional benefit of this dietary/lifestyle program is that it can also help you attain your ideal weight. *The Low-Starch Diabetes Solution* by Dr. Rob Thompson, which promotes the consumption of low glycemic load foods—not low glycemic index—is a clear and powerful demonstration of how eliminating or minimizing the presence of starches in your diet can dramatically improve your health.

Carbohydrates, Fiber and Diabetes Information Resources

1. Anderson, et al, "Carbohydrate and Fiber Recommendations for Individuals with Diabetes: A Quantitative Assessment and Meta-Analysis of the Evidence," Journal of the American College of Nutrition, Vol. 23, No. 1, 5-17 (2004)
2. The Harvard School of Public Health Nutrition Source Newsletter, "Fiber," http://www.hsph.harvard.edu/nutritionsource/what-should-you-eat/fiber/

Reviewed by: **Jay Krakovitz, M.D.,** for:

DIABETES SELF-DEFENSE, LLC
6360 Quail Street, Denver, CO 80004
Cell: 303-931-9710; **Web:** www.DiabetesSelfDefense.com

Week Beginning: _____

Weekly Record

MON:	Time	Bld Sgr	Meals	Net Carbs(g)	2 Hrs Bld Sgr	Blood Press	Exercise/Min	Notes/Sickness
Breakfast								
Lunch								
Dinner								
Bedtime								

TUES:	Time	Bld Sgr	Meals	Net Carbs(g)	2 Hrs Bld Sgr	Blood Press	Exercise/Min	Notes/Sickness
Breakfast								
Lunch								
Dinner								
Bedtime								

WED:	Time	Bld Sgr	Meals	Net Carbs(g)	2 Hrs Bld Sgr	Blood Press	Exercise/Min	Notes/Sickness
Breakfast								
Lunch								
Dinner								
Bedtime								

THUR:	Time	Bld Sgr	Meals	Net Carbs(g)	2 Hrs Bld Sgr	Blood Press	Exercise/Min	Notes/Sickness
Breakfast								
Lunch								
Dinner								
Bedtime								

FRI:	Time	Bld Sgr	Meals	Net Carbs(g)	2 Hrs Bld Sgr	Blood Press	Exercise/Min	Notes/Sickness
Breakfast								
Lunch								
Dinner								
Bedtime								

SAT:	Time	Bld Sgr	Meals	Net Carbs(g)	2 Hrs Bld Sgr	Blood Press	Exercise/Min	Notes/Sickness
Breakfast								
Lunch								
Dinner								
Bedtime								

SUN:	Time	Bld Sgr	Meals	Net Carbs(g)	2 Hrs Bld Sgr	Blood Press	Exercise/Min	Notes/Sickness
Breakfast								
Lunch								
Dinner								
Bedtime								

Week 9:
The Power of Low-Carb Diets

What Does Science Say about Low-Carb Diets and Diabetes?

Three recent articles in the journal *Nutrition and Metabolism* highlight the value of carbohydrate-restriction in the treatment of diabetes and metabolic syndrome. Nielsen, et al. provides a follow-up of a patient study now carried out to forty-four months. *Conclusion*: Advice to obese patients with Type 2 diabetes to follow a 20 percent carbohydrate diet with some caloric restriction has lasting effects on body weight and glycemic control. Moreover, Westman and Vernon suggest that if the aggressive attempt to lower glucose in the ACCORD trials had relied on carbohydrate restriction rather than pharmacology the unexpected deaths that resulted in termination of that part of the study might have been avoided. Westman and Vernon conclude: "The inattention to potent dietary therapy in all recent major diabetes studies, including the recent ACCORD trial, should not lead us to forget about carbohydrate-restriction as a means to achieve weight loss and glycemic control without hypoglycemia."

Why Should I Be Concerned about Low-Carb Diets?

In December 2007, the American Diabetes Association for the first time endorsed the low-carb diet as a viable diet for weight loss. Richard Bernstein, MD, in his book, *The Diabetes Diet*, states that "there should be no more mystery that low-carb is the way to go for people with diabetes." Accurso, et al. represents a summary of the positive effects of carbohydrate restriction and is intended as a constructive alternative to the 2008 nutritional guidelines from the American Diabetes Association (ADA).

Twenty-four authors conclude: Carbohydrate restriction is an intuitive and rational approach to improvement of glycemic and metabolic control. Data demonstrating that weight loss and cardiovascular risk are also improved remove these barriers to the acceptance of carbohydrate restriction as a reasonable if not the preferred treatment for Type 2 diabetes. Finally, carbohydrate restriction is a potentially favorable diet for improving components of the metabolic syndrome and thereby for the prevention of diabetes.

How Can I Create a Customized Low-Carb Diet?

Dr. Bernstein's book, mentioned above, offers a variety of ways for you to create your own low-carb diet, to your personal tastes. Another of the more successful methods for achieving your optimum weight and health is *The Paleo Diet*, an easy-to-follow low-carb program that has had an outstanding track record. A third resource, *The Low-Starch Diabetes Solution* by Rob Thompson, MD, is a well-balanced and easy-to-follow program. Remember to check out the various sources to develop a program that best fits you and your lifestyle.

Low-Carb Diets and Diabetes Information Resources

1. Nielsen JV, Joensson EA: Low-carbohydrate diet in type 2 diabetes: stable improvement of bodyweight and glycemic control during 44 months follow-up. *Nutrition and Metabolism* (Lond) 2008, 5(1):14.
2. Westman EC, Vernon MC: Has carbohydrate-restriction been forgotten as a treatment for diabetes mellitus? A perspective on the ACCORD study design. *Nutrition and Metabolism* (Lond) 2008, 5:10.
3. Accurso A, Bernstein RK, Dahlqvist A, Draznin B, Feinman RD, Fine EJ, Gleed A, Jacobs DB, LarsonG, Lustig RH et al: Dietary carbohydrate restriction in type 2 diabetes mellitus and metabolic syndrome: time for a critical appraisal. *Nutrition andMetabolism* (Lond) 2008, 5(1):9.
4. American Diabetes Association: Nutrition Recommendations and Interventions for Diabetes-2008. *Diabetes Care* 2008, 31(Supplement 1):S61-S78.

Reviewed by: **Jay Krakovitz, M.D.,** for:

DIABETES SELF-DEFENSE, LLC
6360 Quail Street, Denver, CO 80004
Cell: 303-931-9710; **Web:** www.DiabetesSelfDefense.com

Week Beginning: _____

Weekly Record

MON:	Time	Bld Sgr	Meals	Net Carbs(g)	2 Hrs Bld Sgr	Blood Press	Exercise/Min	Notes/Sickness
Breakfast								
Lunch								
Dinner								
Bedtime								

TUES:	Time	Bld Sgr	Meals	Net Carbs(g)	2 Hrs Bld Sgr	Blood Press	Exercise/Min	Notes/Sickness
Breakfast								
Lunch								
Dinner								
Bedtime								

WED:	Time	Bld Sgr	Meals	Net Carbs(g)	2 Hrs Bld Sgr	Blood Press	Exercise/Min	Notes/Sickness
Breakfast								
Lunch								
Dinner								
Bedtime								

THUR:	Time	Bld Sgr	Meals	Net Carbs(g)	2 Hrs Bld Sgr	Blood Press	Exercise/Min	Notes/Sickness
Breakfast								
Lunch								
Dinner								
Bedtime								

FRI:	Time	Bld Sgr	Meals	Net Carbs(g)	2 Hrs Bld Sgr	Blood Press	Exercise/Min	Notes/Sickness
Breakfast								
Lunch								
Dinner								
Bedtime								

SAT:	Time	Bld Sgr	Meals	Net Carbs(g)	2 Hrs Bld Sgr	Blood Press	Exercise/Min	Notes/Sickness
Breakfast								
Lunch								
Dinner								
Bedtime								

SUN:	Time	Bld Sgr	Meals	Net Carbs(g)	2 Hrs Bld Sgr	Blood Press	Exercise/Min	Notes/Sickness
Breakfast								
Lunch								
Dinner								
Bedtime								

Week 10:
Dietary Fats and Oils

What Does Science Say about Dietary Fats, Oils, and Diabetes?

While polyunsaturated and monounsaturated fats are good for health in the right quantities, the primary dietary fat goal in persons with diabetes is to limit saturated fat and trans fatty acid intake. Saturated fat, in general, is the principal dietary determinant of LDL or *bad* cholesterol. Furthermore, persons with diabetes appear to be more sensitive to dietary cholesterol than the general public. In non-diabetic persons, low saturated fat and cholesterol diets decrease total cholesterol, LDL cholesterol, and triglycerides with mixed effects on HDL or *good* cholesterol.

Positive correlations between dietary total and saturated fat and changes in total cholesterol and LDL and HDL cholesterol are observed. Adding exercise results in greater decreases in plasma total and LDL cholesterol and triglycerides and prevents the decrease in HDL cholesterol associated with low-fat diets. However, studies in persons with diabetes demonstrating effects of specific percentages of dietary saturated fatty acids and specific amounts of dietary cholesterol are not available. Therefore, the goal for persons with diabetes remains the same as for the general population in terms of dietary fat consumption.

Where Are Most *Saturated* Fats and *Trans*-Fatty Acids Found?

Saturated fats are found in foods from both animal and vegetable sources. Animal sources include meat, poultry, and whole-milk dairy products such as cheese, milk, ice cream, cream, butter, and lard. Vegetable sources—including coconut, palm kernel, and palm oils—are also high in saturated fat. It is not uncommon to find many sugar-free dessert products loaded with saturated fats! *Trans*-fatty acids (formed when vegetable oils are processed and made more solid ([hydrogenation]), are similar to saturated fats in raising LDL cholesterol. In addition, *trans*-fatty acids lower plasma HDL cholesterol. However, there are some saturated fats—such as those found in coconut oil—that may actually have benefits as pointed out in a recent article by David Mendosa.

Therefore, intake of *trans*-fatty acids should be limited, which includes margarine, salad dressings, fried foods, and bakery products like packaged cakes, cookies, French fries, fried chicken, potato chips, and many processed foods. Remember to read food labels carefully.

So What Are the Guidelines for Fat Consumption from the ADA?

The guidelines for fat consumption from the American Diabetes Association are:

- Less than 10 percent of calorie intake should be derived from saturated fats. Some individuals (i.e., persons with LDL cholesterol greater than or equal to 100 mg/dl) may benefit from lowering saturated fat intake to less than 7 percent of energy intake.
- Dietary cholesterol intake should be less than 300 mg/day. Some individuals (i.e., persons with LDL cholesterol greater than or equal to 100 mg/dl) may benefit from lowering dietary cholesterol to less than 200 mg/ day.
- A low-fat, low-carbohydrate meal plan is recommended to best manage weight and blood fats.
- Intake of *trans*-fatty acids should be minimized as found in many fried foods (fried chicken, French fries) and baked goods (cakes, pies) as well as margarine.

Dietary Fat and Diabetes Information Resources

1. The American Diabetes Association, "Specific Types of Fat" or http://www.diabetes.org/food-and-fitness/food/what-can-i-eat/fat-and-diabetes.html
2. The American Association of Diabetes Educators at www.diabeteseducator.org
3. Mendosa, David, "The Trouble With Saturated Fat," March 12, 2012, http://www.healthcentral.com/diabetes/c/17/150821/trouble-saturated/2?ic=2601

Reviewed by: **Jay Krakovitz, M.D.,** for:

DIABETES SELF-DEFENSE, LLC
6360 Quail Street, Denver, CO 80004
Cell: 303-931-9710; **Web:** www.DiabetesSelfDefense.com

Week Beginning: _____

Weekly Record

MON:	Time	Bld Sgr	Meals	Net Carbs(g)	2 Hrs Bld Sgr	Blood Press	Exercise/Min	Notes/Sickness
Breakfast								
Lunch								
Dinner								
Bedtime								

TUES:	Time	Bld Sgr	Meals	Net Carbs(g)	2 Hrs Bld Sgr	Blood Press	Exercise/Min	Notes/Sickness
Breakfast								
Lunch								
Dinner								
Bedtime								

WED:	Time	Bld Sgr	Meals	Net Carbs(g)	2 Hrs Bld Sgr	Blood Press	Exercise/Min	Notes/Sickness
Breakfast								
Lunch								
Dinner								
Bedtime								

THUR:	Time	Bld Sgr	Meals	Net Carbs(g)	2 Hrs Bld Sgr	Blood Press	Exercise/Min	Notes/Sickness
Breakfast								
Lunch								
Dinner								
Bedtime								

FRI:	Time	Bld Sgr	Meals	Net Carbs(g)	2 Hrs Bld Sgr	Blood Press	Exercise/Min	Notes/Sickness
Breakfast								
Lunch								
Dinner								
Bedtime								

SAT:	Time	Bld Sgr	Meals	Net Carbs(g)	2 Hrs Bld Sgr	Blood Press	Exercise/Min	Notes/Sickness
Breakfast								
Lunch								
Dinner								
Bedtime								

SUN:	Time	Bld Sgr	Meals	Net Carbs(g)	2 Hrs Bld Sgr	Blood Press	Exercise/Min	Notes/Sickness
Breakfast								
Lunch								
Dinner								
Bedtime								

Week 11:
Soy Protein and Diabetes

What Does Science Say about Soy Protein and Diabetes?

Like most dietary matters, there are differing opinions on the value of adding soy or isolated soy protein to the diabetic diet. However, it's now clear that there is scientific evidence to support the incorporation of soy protein into diabetes management. The U.S. Department of Agriculture (USDA) recently stated in a published study that, "In studies of human subjects with or without diabetes, soy protein appears to moderate hyperglycemia (high blood sugar) and reduce body weight, hyperlipidemia (high cholesterol/lipids), and hypersinulinemia (high insulin levels due to high blood sugar), supporting its beneficial effects on obesity and diabetes."

Are All Sources of Soy Protein Equal in Terms of Their Health Benefits for People with Diabetes?

The short answer is no; you need to carefully incorporate soy protein in your diet. While the number of soy products on the shelf at the supermarket is growing rapidly, as are soy dietary supplements, nutritional experts still conclude that the best sources of soy protein are from whole foods like tofu, soybeans, and soy milk.

How Can I Best Incorporate Soy Protein into My Diet?

As with any nutritional component that's being added to your meal plan, incorporate soy products in moderation and balance. For cardiovascular benefits, studies show that you need to consume twenty-five grams or more per day of soy protein, but you don't necessarily need that much to realize other benefits due to its low-fat, low-carb profile. Good sources of natural soy can be found on the shelves in supermarkets and health food stores in the form of tofu, soy milk, soy nuts, soy burgers, and soy puddings. Just be sure to read the label carefully as some commercially prepared soy products can have more harmful ingredients—such as sugars and fats—than healthy ones. Most medical experts recommend that you get your soy from natural foods, not from soy supplements.

Soy Protein and Diabetes Information Resources

1. Teixeira, S. *Journal of Nutrition*, "Soy Supplement Lowers Risk of Common Diabetes Complications," August, 2004; vol 134: pp 1874-1889.
2. *American Journal of Clinical Nutrition* 2002 Dec; 76 (6):1191-201. "Beneficial role of dietary phytoestrogens in obesity and diabetes." Bhathena SJ, Velasquez MT. Phytonutrients Laboratory, Beltsville Human Nutrition Research Center, Agricultural Research Service, US Department of Agriculture, Beltsville, MD 20705, USA.
3. *European Journal of Clinical Nutrition* 2003 Oct; 57 (10):1292-1294. "Beneficiary effect of dietary soy protein on lowering plasma levels of lipid and improving kidney function in type II diabetes with nephropathy." Azadbakht L, et al.
4. *American Journal of Clinical Nutrition* 2002 Dec; 76 (6):1191-201. "Beneficial role of dietary phytoestrogens in obesity and diabetes." Bhathena SJ, Velasquez MT. Phytonutrients Laboratory, Beltsville Human Nutrition Research Center, Agricultural Research Service, US Department of Agriculture, Beltsville, MD 20705, USA.

Reviewed by: **Jay Krakovitz, M.D.,** for:

DIABETES SELF-DEFENSE, LLC
6360 Quail Street, Denver, CO 80004
Cell: 303-931-9710; **Web:** www.DiabetesSelfDefense.com

Week Beginning: _____

Weekly Record

MON:	Time	Bld Sgr	Meals	Net Carbs(g)	2 Hrs Bld Sgr	Blood Press	Exercise/Min	Notes/Sickness
Breakfast								
Lunch								
Dinner								
Bedtime								

TUES:	Time	Bld Sgr	Meals	Net Carbs(g)	2 Hrs Bld Sgr	Blood Press	Exercise/Min	Notes/Sickness
Breakfast								
Lunch								
Dinner								
Bedtime								

WED:	Time	Bld Sgr	Meals	Net Carbs(g)	2 Hrs Bld Sgr	Blood Press	Exercise/Min	Notes/Sickness
Breakfast								
Lunch								
Dinner								
Bedtime								

THUR:	Time	Bld Sgr	Meals	Net Carbs(g)	2 Hrs Bld Sgr	Blood Press	Exercise/Min	Notes/Sickness
Breakfast								
Lunch								
Dinner								
Bedtime								

FRI:	Time	Bld Sgr	Meals	Net Carbs(g)	2 Hrs Bld Sgr	Blood Press	Exercise/Min	Notes/Sickness
Breakfast								
Lunch								
Dinner								
Bedtime								

SAT:	Time	Bld Sgr	Meals	Net Carbs(g)	2 Hrs Bld Sgr	Blood Press	Exercise/Min	Notes/Sickness
Breakfast								
Lunch								
Dinner								
Bedtime								

SUN:	Time	Bld Sgr	Meals	Net Carbs(g)	2 Hrs Bld Sgr	Blood Press	Exercise/Min	Notes/Sickness
Breakfast								
Lunch								
Dinner								
Bedtime								

Week 12:
The Best Beverages for People with Diabetes

What Does Science Say about the Best Beverages for People with Diabetes?

In general, the recommendations for the general public, when it comes to which beverages or liquids are best to consume on a regular basis, are exactly the same for people with diabetes in a beverage pyramid: (1) water as the foundation (up to nine servings); (2) unsweetened tea and coffee (four to eight servings); (3) low-fat, skim, and soy milk (two servings); (4) non-calorie or diet drinks (four servings); (5) caloric drinks with some nutrients, such as fruit juices, full-fat milk or sports drinks (one serving); and (6) calorically sweetened drinks such as soft drinks (1 serving).

While the major thing that people with diabetes have to watch with beverage consumption—just like with food consumption—is the carbohydrate content of their beverages, they also need to incorporate beverage carbs into their meal plans just like regular foods. Recent studies have shown that, in the USA, adults on average consume 21 percent of their daily calories in the form of drinks.

A major study published in 2008 in the *Archives of Internal Medicine* (*Arch Intern Med.* 2008;168(14):1487-1492) on sugar-sweetened beverages among African American women showed that when high levels of soft drinks or fruit drinks were consumed, there was an increased risk of Type 2 diabetes. Therefore, caution is key with all sugar-sweetened drinks.

Why Should I Be Concerned about Beverage Consumption?

When it comes to beverage consumption, not including water or diet soda that is calorie-free, people with diabetes have to understand that liquids are digested and absorbed into the bloodstream much more quickly than regular carbohydrates that are broken down in the digestive tract. Therefore, high calorie beverages that are consumed in between meals have the potential to create abnormally high and unsafe blood sugar levels; the best general advice is to consume beverages with calories during your regular meal occasions. If you are insulin-dependent, it is even more critical to make sure you account for all beverage carbohydrates and consume them with your meal. On the other hand, certain beverages like milk, regular soft drinks, and orange juice, when taken in half-cup servings, can be a useful tool for correcting low blood sugar or hypoglycemia; just be careful not to overdo it.

How Can I Choose My Beverages Wisely?

Water is by far the best beverage of choice, whether one is diabetic or non-diabetic. Green and black teas have been found to offer significant antioxidant properties, as has coffee, and even an occasional glass of wine can be beneficial. Choosing your beverages wisely and incorporating them into your diabetes meal plan with careful attention to carbohydrate content is still the best advice around. While diet sodas and many flavored waters offer calorie-free options, you will want to only consume them in moderation as the jury is still out on the long-term of effects of their sweetening agents such as Splenda® (sucralose), NutraSweet® (aspartame), and saccharin, even though these sweeteners are FDA-approved. Bottled waters have not been scientifically proven to offer any health benefits over garden-variety tap water, but the choice is up to you.

Diabetes Beverage Information Resources

1. *The Healthy Beverage Guidelines: a Tool to Fight Obesity*, International Diabetes Federation (http://www.idf.org/articles/the-healthy-beverage-guidelines-a-tool-to-fight-obesity), December, 2006.
2. "*Diabetes Bars and Beverages: The Benefits and the Controversies,*" *Diabetes Spectrum* 15: 11-14, 2002 © American Diabetes Association.

Reviewed by: **Jay Krakovitz, M.D.,** for:

DIABETES SELF-DEFENSE, LLC
6360 Quail Street, Denver, CO 80004
Cell: 303-931-9710; **Web:** www.DiabetesSelfDefense.com

Week Beginning: _____

Weekly Record

MON:	Time	Bld Sgr	Meals	Net Carbs(g)	2 Hrs Bld Sgr	Blood Press	Exercise/Min	Notes/Sickness
Breakfast								
Lunch								
Dinner								
Bedtime								

TUES:	Time	Bld Sgr	Meals	Net Carbs(g)	2 Hrs Bld Sgr	Blood Press	Exercise/Min	Notes/Sickness
Breakfast								
Lunch								
Dinner								
Bedtime								

WED:	Time	Bld Sgr	Meals	Net Carbs(g)	2 Hrs Bld Sgr	Blood Press	Exercise/Min	Notes/Sickness
Breakfast								
Lunch								
Dinner								
Bedtime								

THUR:	Time	Bld Sgr	Meals	Net Carbs(g)	2 Hrs Bld Sgr	Blood Press	Exercise/Min	Notes/Sickness
Breakfast								
Lunch								
Dinner								
Bedtime								

FRI:	Time	Bld Sgr	Meals	Net Carbs(g)	2 Hrs Bld Sgr	Blood Press	Exercise/Min	Notes/Sickness
Breakfast								
Lunch								
Dinner								
Bedtime								

SAT:	Time	Bld Sgr	Meals	Net Carbs(g)	2 Hrs Bld Sgr	Blood Press	Exercise/Min	Notes/Sickness
Breakfast								
Lunch								
Dinner								
Bedtime								

SUN:	Time	Bld Sgr	Meals	Net Carbs(g)	2 Hrs Bld Sgr	Blood Press	Exercise/Min	Notes/Sickness
Breakfast								
Lunch								
Dinner								
Bedtime								

Week 13:
Antioxidants and Diabetes

What Does Science Say about Antioxidant Foods and Diabetes?

Eating a colorful diet full of antioxidant-rich fruits and vegetables may help prevent diabetes. A new study shows that people whose diets had the highest levels vitamin E were 30 percent less likely to develop Type 2 diabetes than those who ate the least amounts of the antioxidants. In addition, researchers found that people who ate a lot of carotenoids, a type of antioxidant found in colorful fruits and vegetables, also had a lower risk of developing Type 2 diabetes.

But the study showed one of the most popular antioxidants, vitamin C, seemed to offer no protection against the disease. Antioxidants are found in whole grains, fruits, and vegetables. Previous research has suggested that eating a diet rich in these compounds can have a variety of healthy effects, such as preventing chronic diseases like diabetes, by fighting free radicals, unstable molecules that cause cell damage within the body.

Will Eating Foods Rich in Antioxidants Help Me—If I Am Already Diabetic?

According to James Anderson, MD, professor of medicine and clinical nutrition at the University of Kentucky in Lexington, antioxidant vitamins like vitamins C and E attained through diet are extraordinarily important for the diabetic patient.

"Most evidence suggests a higher fiber diet rich in whole grains, fruits, and vegetables, and lower fat," according to Dr. Anderson. Natural foods rich in vitamin E include almonds, peanut butter, margarine, wheat germ, sunflower oil, kiwi, broccoli, and eggs. Vitamin C-rich foods include papaya, orange juice, strawberries, cantaloupe, green peppers, broccoli, and tomatoes. Fruits, vegetables, and whole-grains like barley and oats are natural and plentiful sources of antioxidant vitamins.

What about Antioxidant Supplements—Are They Supported by Science?

Heart disease causes more than 70 percent of deaths in people with diabetes, according to Ishwarial Jialal, PhD, professor of internal medicine and pathology and co-director of the Lipid Clinic at the University of Texas Southwestern Medical Center at Dallas.

"The diabetics' risk for heart disease is so great, it's [a good idea] to take an antioxidant supplement because it not only functions as an antioxidant, but anti-inflammatory [as well]," he says. However, the 2004 American Heart Association science advisory on the subject of antioxidant vitamins and cardiovascular disease asserted that there is insufficient evidence to justify the use of antioxidant vitamins for cardiovascular risk reduction. It is best to get your antioxidants through your diet.

Antioxidants and Diabetes Information Resources

1. Montonen, J. "Antioxidant Foods and Diabetes," *Diabetes Care*, February 2004; vol. 27: pp362-366.
2. WebMD Medical News Archive, "Heart Disease and Antioxidants, Vitamin E and Beta-Carotene, at http://www.webmd.com/heart-disease/guide/antioxidants-vitamin-e
3. www.wholehealthmd.com *"Your Antioxidant Cocktail,"* at http://www.wholehealthmd.com/ME2/dirmod.asp?sid=F4B4130C2BD847ACBFDEA959133627F5&nm=Healing+Kitchen&type=AWHN_News&mod=News+Perspectives&tier=3&id=A905A64E16D54CF9828FCA776E533D72

Reviewed by: **Jay Krakovitz, M.D.,** for:

DIABETES SELF-DEFENSE, LLC
6360 Quail Street, Denver, CO 80004
Cell: 303-931-9710; **Web:** www.DiabetesSelfDefense.com

Week Beginning: _____

Weekly Record

MON:	Time	Bld Sgr	Meals	Net Carbs(g)	2 Hrs Bld Sgr	Blood Press	Exercise/Min	Notes/Sickness
Breakfast								
Lunch								
Dinner								
Bedtime								

TUES:	Time	Bld Sgr	Meals	Net Carbs(g)	2 Hrs Bld Sgr	Blood Press	Exercise/Min	Notes/Sickness
Breakfast								
Lunch								
Dinner								
Bedtime								

WED:	Time	Bld Sgr	Meals	Net Carbs(g)	2 Hrs Bld Sgr	Blood Press	Exercise/Min	Notes/Sickness
Breakfast								
Lunch								
Dinner								
Bedtime								

THUR:	Time	Bld Sgr	Meals	Net Carbs(g)	2 Hrs Bld Sgr	Blood Press	Exercise/Min	Notes/Sickness
Breakfast								
Lunch								
Dinner								
Bedtime								

FRI:	Time	Bld Sgr	Meals	Net Carbs(g)	2 Hrs Bld Sgr	Blood Press	Exercise/Min	Notes/Sickness
Breakfast								
Lunch								
Dinner								
Bedtime								

SAT:	Time	Bld Sgr	Meals	Net Carbs(g)	2 Hrs Bld Sgr	Blood Press	Exercise/Min	Notes/Sickness
Breakfast								
Lunch								
Dinner								
Bedtime								

SUN:	Time	Bld Sgr	Meals	Net Carbs(g)	2 Hrs Bld Sgr	Blood Press	Exercise/Min	Notes/Sickness
Breakfast								
Lunch								
Dinner								
Bedtime								

Week 14:
The Glycemic Index and Glycemic Load Concepts

What Is the Glycemic Index and Is It Supported by Science?

Some of the popular media and self-help books have been promoting the "glycemic index" as a tool for helping to manage blood glucose levels. Glycemic index, or GI, is a measurement of the effect that a food has on blood glucose—specifically the ability of a food to raise blood sugar levels within two to three hours after eating. It applies mainly to carbohydrates. Health columns in numerous publications have listed foods with "high" or "low" GI as a guide for helping to balance carbohydrate intake. The American Diabetes Association (ADA), however, in its recently released nutritional guidelines, concludes that the GI is not an appropriate guide for people with diabetes.

ADA's experts scrutinized existing research studies on the effects of high GI diets versus low GI diets in Type 2 diabetes. They found that a high GI diet had no adverse effect on measures of blood glucose or cholesterol. They also found that a low GI diet provided no convincing evidence of long-term benefit. These findings led to the ADA's conclusion that the total amount of carbohydrates eaten rather than the type determines the blood sugar response.

Should I Be Concerned about the Glycemic Index of the Foods I Eat?

As a diabetic who has personally experimented with high and low glycemic foods, I have found in my experience that low GI foods like barley, beans, and soy milk can be quite beneficial in the diabetic diet. There are many doctors like Julian Whitaker, MD, author of *Reversing Diabetes*, that have had good results in recommending low GI diets, and some studies have shown positive results with a low GI diet. So while it probably can't hurt, you don't necessarily need to get too caught up with it beyond using it as yet one more tool in the War Against Diabetes; learn which of your favorite foods have low GIs, and eat them often within your diet plan. By tracking your sugars, you will discover how helpful a low GI diet is for your unique situation.

What Is the Glycemic Load Concept...and Is It Supported by Science?

To understand how a carbohydrate food affects your blood sugar, you need to know both its ranking on the glycemic index and how many grams of carbohydrate a normal serving contains. This measure is the *glycemic load*, which can be calculated by multiplying the carbohydrate content per serving by the food's glycemic index number. Although you'll see glycemic index rankings written as whole numbers, they actually are percentages, so if the GI of a food is 71, treat this as 71 percent when you multiply it by the grams of carbohydrate in a serving.

Foods with a low glycemic load rank from 1 to 10; those with medium load range from 11-19 and those with high glycemic load rank at 20 or above. Judging from their high glycemic index—up to 97 in some studies—carrots would seem to be a food to avoid if you are carbohydrate sensitive. A half-cup serving of carrots contains only 6.2 grams of carbs, so the glycemic load of that portion would be 6.2 x 97%—or 6, a low value. By contrast, a plain 5-ounce bagel provides 65 grams of carbohydrate and has a GI of 71. Its glycemic load (65 x 72%) is a whopping 47. The ADA does not at this time endorse the glycemic load concept, but again, you may find it useful in your case.

Some of the best books recently published on understanding the difference between the Glycemic Index and the Glycemic Load and how to develop improved nutritional strategies for people with diabetes are from Rob Thompson, MD, and include *The Low-Starch Diabetes Solution* and *The Sugar Blockers Diet*.

The Glycemic Index/Glycemic Load Information Resources

1. American Diabetes Association, "Evidence-based nutritional principles and recommendations for the treatment and prevention of diabetes and related complications." *Diabetes Care*, January 2002; 25:202.
2. Palu M, United States Potato Board. "New dietary guidelines from the ADA address glycemic index." March 22, 2002.
3. Mendosa, David, A Writer on the Web, http://www.mendosa.com/gilists.htm
4. Thompson, Rob, MD, *The Low-Starch Diabetes Solution*, © 2010 Robert Thompson, MD

Reviewed by: **Jay Krakovitz, M.D.,** for:

DIABETES SELF-DEFENSE, LLC
6360 Quail Street, Denver, CO 80004
Cell: 303-931-9710; **Web:** www.DiabetesSelfDefense.com

Week Beginning: _____

Weekly Record

MON:	Time	Bld Sgr	Meals	Net Carbs(g)	2 Hrs Bld Sgr	Blood Press	Exercise/Min	Notes/Sickness
Breakfast								
Lunch								
Dinner								
Bedtime								

TUES:	Time	Bld Sgr	Meals	Net Carbs(g)	2 Hrs Bld Sgr	Blood Press	Exercise/Min	Notes/Sickness
Breakfast								
Lunch								
Dinner								
Bedtime								

WED:	Time	Bld Sgr	Meals	Net Carbs(g)	2 Hrs Bld Sgr	Blood Press	Exercise/Min	Notes/Sickness
Breakfast								
Lunch								
Dinner								
Bedtime								

THUR:	Time	Bld Sgr	Meals	Net Carbs(g)	2 Hrs Bld Sgr	Blood Press	Exercise/Min	Notes/Sickness
Breakfast								
Lunch								
Dinner								
Bedtime								

FRI:	Time	Bld Sgr	Meals	Net Carbs(g)	2 Hrs Bld Sgr	Blood Press	Exercise/Min	Notes/Sickness
Breakfast								
Lunch								
Dinner								
Bedtime								

SAT:	Time	Bld Sgr	Meals	Net Carbs(g)	2 Hrs Bld Sgr	Blood Press	Exercise/Min	Notes/Sickness
Breakfast								
Lunch								
Dinner								
Bedtime								

SUN:	Time	Bld Sgr	Meals	Net Carbs(g)	2 Hrs Bld Sgr	Blood Press	Exercise/Min	Notes/Sickness
Breakfast								
Lunch								
Dinner								
Bedtime								

Week 15:
Dining Out and Diabetes

What Are the Most Important Facts about Dining Out and Diabetes?

Thanks in large part to the growing health trend in the United States, more and more restaurants are offering healthier options for their customers, thereby making it much easier to eat healthy. Even fast food outlets like McDonald's and Wendy's today offer items like salads, low-calorie salad dressings, grilled chicken sandwiches, and milk instead of soda. Traditional restaurants are also stepping up to the plate and offering low-carb and low-fat lunches and dinners.

Nevertheless, it is still critical for the person with diabetes to choose wisely when dining out. Nutritional information may or may not be readily available, so it is always best to choose foods that are low in sugar, fat, and sodium, and most of the time this means items that have been baked, grilled, or steamed—but not fried. Restaurants and fast food outlets also still tend to serve large portion sizes, so never feel embarrassed about eating only half of the food served and taking the rest home for later consumption.

Eating smaller portions applies to desserts as well, even if you order a traditional dessert and eat only a few bites, like a small portion of pumpkin pie. Like anything else in diabetes management, it's up to you to carefully monitor and manage the foods you eat—because people with diabetes each know their own individual meal plans based on their individual preferences, medications, and activity levels.

If I Have Diabetes, Should I Be Concerned about Dining Out Occasionally?

In general, you shouldn't have to worry any more than when you normally eat. The American Diabetes Association (ADA) recommends that you plan ahead when dining out in order the make the best choices for your unique needs and to eat fruits, whole grains, and vegetables as much as possible, even at restaurants. You should always feel free to tell the waiter that you have diabetes and to ask if they can accommodate any of your special requests. Remember to minimize the amount of corn, cereal grains, breads, pasta, potatoes, and rice—all of which are high in starch.

How Can I Eat "Diabetes Healthy" When Dining Out?

When you eat out, order only what you need and want. Know how to make changes in your meal plan in case the restaurant doesn't have just what you want. Some helpful guidelines include these suggestions from the ADA: (1) If you don't know what's in a dish, ask;(2) Try to eat the same portion you would at home; (3) Eat slowly; (4) Ask for fish or meat to be broiled with no extra butter; (5) Order your baked potato plain, then top it with a teaspoon of margarine or low-calorie sour cream; (6) Ask for food to be prepared without added salt or MSG; (7) Ask for sauces, gravies or salad dressings "on the side" and use sparingly; (8) Do not order any fried foods like fried chicken/nuggets, fried fish or French fries; and (9) Limit alcohol intake to no more than one drink.

Dining Out and Diabetes Information Resources

1. The American Diabetes Association, "Your Guide to Eating Out" at 1-800-342-2383 or http://www.diabetes.org/food-and-fitness/food/what-can-i-eat/eating-out/
2. The Canadian Diabetes Association, "A Guide To Eating Out," at 1-800-226-8464 or http://www.diabetes.ca/diabetes-and-you/nutrition/eating-out/

Reviewed by: **Jay Krakovitz, M.D.,** for:

DIABETES SELF-DEFENSE, LLC
6360 Quail Street, Denver, CO 80004
Cell: 303-931-9710; **Web:** www.DiabetesSelfDefense.com

Week Beginning: _____

Weekly Record

MON:	Time	Bld Sgr	Meals	Net Carbs(g)	2 Hrs Bld Sgr	Blood Press	Exercise/Min	Notes/Sickness
Breakfast								
Lunch								
Dinner								
Bedtime								

TUES:	Time	Bld Sgr	Meals	Net Carbs(g)	2 Hrs Bld Sgr	Blood Press	Exercise/Min	Notes/Sickness
Breakfast								
Lunch								
Dinner								
Bedtime								

WED:	Time	Bld Sgr	Meals	Net Carbs(g)	2 Hrs Bld Sgr	Blood Press	Exercise/Min	Notes/Sickness
Breakfast								
Lunch								
Dinner								
Bedtime								

THUR:	Time	Bld Sgr	Meals	Net Carbs(g)	2 Hrs Bld Sgr	Blood Press	Exercise/Min	Notes/Sickness
Breakfast								
Lunch								
Dinner								
Bedtime								

FRI:	Time	Bld Sgr	Meals	Net Carbs(g)	2 Hrs Bld Sgr	Blood Press	Exercise/Min	Notes/Sickness
Breakfast								
Lunch								
Dinner								
Bedtime								

SAT:	Time	Bld Sgr	Meals	Net Carbs(g)	2 Hrs Bld Sgr	Blood Press	Exercise/Min	Notes/Sickness
Breakfast								
Lunch								
Dinner								
Bedtime								

SUN:	Time	Bld Sgr	Meals	Net Carbs(g)	2 Hrs Bld Sgr	Blood Press	Exercise/Min	Notes/Sickness
Breakfast								
Lunch								
Dinner								
Bedtime								

Week 16:
Diabetes and Medical Nutrition Therapy

What Does Science Say about Diabetes and Medical Nutrition Therapy?

While no one denies the value of *medical nutrition therapy* (MNT) from a registered dietitian, there has historically been little data to relate it to glycemic or blood sugar control. Now, however, research reported at a recent American Diabetes Association (ADA) meeting provides data showing that patients who received MNT from a dietitian showed *much greater improvement in A1C* than those who did not. Researchers conducted a chart review of 162 adults with diabetes from nine ambulatory health centers in an integrated healthcare network.

The network serves a multi-ethnic, indigent patient population; more than 60 percent of the patients whose charts were reviewed did not speak English. The study found that those patients who had had at least two visits with a registered dietitian during the year studied reduced their HbA1c by 20 percent, bringing mean levels to 8 percent. Only 2.2 percent of these patients needed to increase or add diabetes medication during the study period. In comparison, subjects without MNT education had a 2 percent decline in HbA1c, with mean levels remaining above 8 percent. Thus, the researchers reported, MNT by registered dietitians is an essential and effective component in the management of adult patients with diabetes in multicultural outpatient settings.

Does Medicare Cover Medical Nutrition Therapy?

Medicare Part B now covers medical nutrition therapy for all people with diabetes. Coverage was previously limited to those with uncontrolled diabetes and those who were on kidney dialysis. Now, an estimated 4.5 million Medicare recipients plus more than one hundred thousand people with kidney disease are eligible for individualized medical nutrition therapy that will help teach them how to eat better to control their diseases or to lose weight. The change came about after a government-sponsored study showed that nutrition counseling with a dietitian is cost-effective, with the greatest impact in people with diabetes and kidney disease.

Instead of paying for the costly consequences of poor nutrition, the government recognized the benefit in paying for services that may well prevent the complications. The new benefit permits people to meet one-on-one with a registered dietitian to discuss diet and exercise, review lab tests, and set goals for making changes in diet. A final decision on the number of such visits is still pending, but a Medicare spokesman estimated that three to four such visits a year would be covered. The new benefits took effect on January 1, 2002. A spokesman for the Centers for Medicare and Medicaid Services (CMS), the federal agency that operates Medicare, told lifeclinic.com, "We are accepting and paying claims now."

Medical Nutrition Therapy Information Resources

1. Johnson EQ, Thomas M., "Medical nutrition therapy by registered dietitians improves HbA1c levels," Presentation at ADA meeting, June 23, 2001. (Abs.)
2. Centers for Medicare and Medicaid Services, "CMS announces physician pay changes for 2002—Final rule expands coverage for preventive services," *Medicare News Release*, Oct. 31, 2001
3. www.medicare.gov, Medical Nutrition Therapy at http://www.medicare.gov/(X(1) S(xfpzk1ffgsblbg45luvjxn55))/navigation/manage-your-health/preventive-services/medical-nutrition-therapy.aspx

Part 4:
"A" = Achieve Common Sense Weight Loss and Fitness Goals

"A" Section Summary

The vast majority of people diagnosed with diabetes are obese or overweight. This happens as a result of more calories going in than are being burned over time with the excess energy being stored as fat. Regardless of the cause, it is vital to provide people with diabetes a "real-world" solution that can be implemented in their everyday lives—forget the fad diets and daily trips to the gym. Scientific studies have shown that only a modest weight loss—5 percent to 7 percent—along with a healthy lifestyle can help people with diabetes gain better control of their blood sugar, blood pressure, and cholesterol. The solution here is not some "magic diet" or "miracle fitness" program but instead a practical, easy-to-follow diet and exercise program that produces real long-term results. One of the more surprising recent research findings is that something as simple as walking at a moderate pace, where you can carry on a normal conversation—not heavy workouts at the gym—for thirty minutes or so every other day can do wonders for improving insulin sensitivity.

Reviewed by: **Jay Krakovitz, M.D.,** for:

DIABETES SELF-DEFENSE, LLC
6360 Quail Street, Denver, CO 80004
Cell: 303-931-9710; **Web:** www.DiabetesSelfDefense.com

Week Beginning: _____

Weekly Record

MON:	Time	Bld Sgr	Meals	Net Carbs(g)	2 Hrs Bld Sgr	Blood Press	Exercise/Min	Notes/Sickness
Breakfast								
Lunch								
Dinner								
Bedtime								

TUES:	Time	Bld Sgr	Meals	Net Carbs(g)	2 Hrs Bld Sgr	Blood Press	Exercise/Min	Notes/Sickness
Breakfast								
Lunch								
Dinner								
Bedtime								

WED:	Time	Bld Sgr	Meals	Net Carbs(g)	2 Hrs Bld Sgr	Blood Press	Exercise/Min	Notes/Sickness
Breakfast								
Lunch								
Dinner								
Bedtime								

THUR:	Time	Bld Sgr	Meals	Net Carbs(g)	2 Hrs Bld Sgr	Blood Press	Exercise/Min	Notes/Sickness
Breakfast								
Lunch								
Dinner								
Bedtime								

FRI:	Time	Bld Sgr	Meals	Net Carbs(g)	2 Hrs Bld Sgr	Blood Press	Exercise/Min	Notes/Sickness
Breakfast								
Lunch								
Dinner								
Bedtime								

SAT:	Time	Bld Sgr	Meals	Net Carbs(g)	2 Hrs Bld Sgr	Blood Press	Exercise/Min	Notes/Sickness
Breakfast								
Lunch								
Dinner								
Bedtime								

SUN:	Time	Bld Sgr	Meals	Net Carbs(g)	2 Hrs Bld Sgr	Blood Press	Exercise/Min	Notes/Sickness
Breakfast								
Lunch								
Dinner								
Bedtime								

Week 17:
Weight Control in Diabetes Management

What Does Science Say about the Relationship Between Weight Control and Diabetes?

Obesity is today considered the primary risk factor for development of diabetes, and excessive calorie intake is a major contributor to poor glycemic control in people that already have Type 2 diabetes. Up to 90 percent of diabetics are estimated to be obese or overweight when first diagnosed with diabetes. People are considered overweight if their Body Mass Index (BMI) is 25-29 and obese if it's 30 or higher. The BMI simply measures the relationship of your height to your current body weight.

After reviewing hundreds of clinical trials on weight loss and diabetes, Dr. James Anderson of the University of the Kentucky College of Medicine concluded that the reviewed data suggest that US health care providers should endorse the American Heart Association's and European diabetes associations' recommendations that diabetic persons achieve and maintain a BMI of less than or equal to 25. *Weight management may be the most important therapeutic task for most obese Type 2 diabetic individuals.*

At the same time, it's important to recognize that 90 percent of people who go on "diets"—whether it's a fad diet or not—fail to keep the weight off in the long-run (five years or more). But the good news is that 10 percent of all dieters have been able to lose weight and keep it off by simply lowering their daily calorie intake to an appropriate level (1200-1800 calories per day, depending on body size) and combining that with adequate daily activity or exercise.

Why Should I Be Concerned about Weight Control?

If you are overweight, your body does not use insulin well. This is called insulin resistance. Even a weight loss of only 5 percent to 7 percent can improve blood sugar control. Weight loss will also lower blood pressure. After weight loss, you may need less diabetes and blood pressure medications, and that saves money. Weight loss relieves pressure on arthritic joints. Most people also have more energy and feel better. You do not have to reduce down to your ideal body weight to see these results. Even if you cannot lose weight, not gaining weight will help. Any change in eating or activity that lowers your blood sugar usually improves your health and fitness level.

How Can I Better Control My Weight?

There are two basic facts about permanent weight loss that you need to be aware of: (1) Weight loss only occurs when calories out (burned) exceed calories in (eating and drinking); and (2) no one can lose weight and keep it off permanently without increasing their physical activity level. One of the more successful methods for permanent weight loss is *The Paleo Diet,* an easy-to-follow program that has had an outstanding track record. You can also get information on weight control as listed below from the National Institute for Diabetes and Digestive and Kidney Disorders (NIDDK) as well as the American Diabetes Association's Program, "Weight Loss Matters." In the end, you need to find and apply the principles of the program that best suits your lifestyle and is the easiest for you to maintain on a long-term basis.

Weight Control and Diabetes Information Resources

1. The National Institute for Diabetes and Digestive and Kidney Disorders at www.niddk.nih.gov/health/nutrit/nutrit.htm
2. The American Diabetes Association at www.diabetes.org/food-and-fitness/fitness/weight-loss/

Reviewed by: **Jay Krakovitz, M.D.,** for:

DIABETES SELF-DEFENSE, LLC
6360 Quail Street, Denver, CO 80004
Cell: 303-931-9710; **Web:** www.DiabetesSelfDefense.com

Week Beginning: _____

Weekly Record

MON:	Time	Bld Sgr	Meals	Net Carbs(g)	2 Hrs Bld Sgr	Blood Press	Exercise/Min	Notes/Sickness
Breakfast								
Lunch								
Dinner								
Bedtime								

TUES:	Time	Bld Sgr	Meals	Net Carbs(g)	2 Hrs Bld Sgr	Blood Press	Exercise/Min	Notes/Sickness
Breakfast								
Lunch								
Dinner								
Bedtime								

WED:	Time	Bld Sgr	Meals	Net Carbs(g)	2 Hrs Bld Sgr	Blood Press	Exercise/Min	Notes/Sickness
Breakfast								
Lunch								
Dinner								
Bedtime								

THUR:	Time	Bld Sgr	Meals	Net Carbs(g)	2 Hrs Bld Sgr	Blood Press	Exercise/Min	Notes/Sickness
Breakfast								
Lunch								
Dinner								
Bedtime								

FRI:	Time	Bld Sgr	Meals	Net Carbs(g)	2 Hrs Bld Sgr	Blood Press	Exercise/Min	Notes/Sickness
Breakfast								
Lunch								
Dinner								
Bedtime								

SAT:	Time	Bld Sgr	Meals	Net Carbs(g)	2 Hrs Bld Sgr	Blood Press	Exercise/Min	Notes/Sickness
Breakfast								
Lunch								
Dinner								
Bedtime								

SUN:	Time	Bld Sgr	Meals	Net Carbs(g)	2 Hrs Bld Sgr	Blood Press	Exercise/Min	Notes/Sickness
Breakfast								
Lunch								
Dinner								
Bedtime								

Week 18:
The Paleo Diet for Weight Control and Optimum Health

What Is the *Paleo Diet*…and Is It Supported by Science?

The Paleo Diet is a simple, easy-to-follow, and highly successful program for better weight and diabetes control, including permanent weight loss, that is built around foods that were eaten by our Paleolithic (Old Stone Age) ancestors. More of a lifestyle versus being a traditional diet, it is based on over twenty-five years of scientific research by Loren Cordain, PhD, at Colorado State University in Fort Collins, Colorado. *The Paleo Diet* has proven itself to be scientifically sound and safe for people with diabetes. In fact, it is a naturally low-carb diet that Dr. Cordain specifically recommends for people with diabetes, both Type 1 and Type 2.

The nutritional guidelines for *The Paleo Diet*, as seen below, make it virtually unnecessary to count grams of carbohydrates, fats, and protein or exchanges—unlike traditional diabetes meal plans. Instead, by simply following *The Paleo Diet* most of the time, your body will gradually and naturally reach its ideal weight while being supplied with optimum nutrition for optimum health. While there are other scientifically-supported diets for people with diabetes like *Dr. Bernstein's Diabetes Solution* by Dr. Richard Bernstein and *The Low-Starch Diabetes Solution* by Rob Thompson, MD, both of which should be investigated to see if they're right for you, the evidence today is overwhelmingly in favor of the low-carb approach as the best possible strategy for control of weight, blood sugar, blood pressure, and cholesterol.

What Are the Specific Nutritional Guidelines of the *Paleo Diet?*

The beauty of *The Paleo Diet* is that you can develop a meal plan with your nutritionist that is specific to your unique dietary and activity preferences—to help ensure you enjoy, stick with, and benefit from the program. While built around the consumption of *lean meats, seafood, fruits, non-starchy vegetables, and nuts/seeds*, with *The Paleo Diet* you can develop your own meal plan based on the foods and recipes you enjoy most. To keep things simple, there are only seven basic rules to follow based on Dr. Cordain's twenty-five-plus years of diet and exercise research:

1. Eat more animal protein than is normally recommended—from lean meats and seafood.
2. Eat only good carbs from fruits and non-starchy vegetables—avoid whole grains, breads, potatoes, pasta, dairy, starchy vegetables, and legumes/beans while minimizing refined sugars.
3. Eat a high-fiber diet—mostly from nuts, fruits and vegetables, not whole grains.
4. Eat mostly good fats—monounsaturated and polyunsaturated, minimizing saturated and trans fats, making sure you get an adequate amount of Omega-3 fats (fish, fish oil, etc.).
5. Eat a high potassium, low sodium diet, which comes naturally from a diet rich in fruits and vegetables.
6. Eat a diet that forms a net alkaline load, which comes naturally from fruits and vegetables.
7. Eat foods that are rich in plant phytochemicals, vitamins, minerals, and antioxidants, which again comes naturally from fruits and vegetables.

If your diabetes healthcare professional is not familiar with *The Paleo Diet*, encourage them to contact Dr. Cordain directly at Colorado State University through his email (Loren.Cordain@ColoState.edu).

The Paleo Diet Information Resources

1. Cordain, Loren, Ph.D., *The Paleo Diet*, ©2002, John Wiley and Sons, Inc. or www.thepaleodiet.com
2. Cordain, Loren, Ph.D., Colorado State University Health Sciences Center, Loren.Cordain@ColoState.edu
3. Thompson, Rob, MD, *The Low-Starch Diabetes Solution*, © 2010 Robert Thompson, MD, www.amazon.com

Reviewed by: **Jay Krakovitz, M.D.,** for:

DIABETES SELF-DEFENSE, LLC
6360 Quail Street, Denver, CO 80004
Cell: 303-931-9710; **Web:** www.DiabetesSelfDefense.com

Week Beginning: _____

Weekly Record

MON:	Time	Bld Sgr	Meals	Net Carbs(g)	2 Hrs Bld Sgr	Blood Press	Exercise/Min	Notes/Sickness
Breakfast								
Lunch								
Dinner								
Bedtime								

TUES:	Time	Bld Sgr	Meals	Net Carbs(g)	2 Hrs Bld Sgr	Blood Press	Exercise/Min	Notes/Sickness
Breakfast								
Lunch								
Dinner								
Bedtime								

WED:	Time	Bld Sgr	Meals	Net Carbs(g)	2 Hrs Bld Sgr	Blood Press	Exercise/Min	Notes/Sickness
Breakfast								
Lunch								
Dinner								
Bedtime								

THUR:	Time	Bld Sgr	Meals	Net Carbs(g)	2 Hrs Bld Sgr	Blood Press	Exercise/Min	Notes/Sickness
Breakfast								
Lunch								
Dinner								
Bedtime								

FRI:	Time	Bld Sgr	Meals	Net Carbs(g)	2 Hrs Bld Sgr	Blood Press	Exercise/Min	Notes/Sickness
Breakfast								
Lunch								
Dinner								
Bedtime								

SAT:	Time	Bld Sgr	Meals	Net Carbs(g)	2 Hrs Bld Sgr	Blood Press	Exercise/Min	Notes/Sickness
Breakfast								
Lunch								
Dinner								
Bedtime								

SUN:	Time	Bld Sgr	Meals	Net Carbs(g)	2 Hrs Bld Sgr	Blood Press	Exercise/Min	Notes/Sickness
Breakfast								
Lunch								
Dinner								
Bedtime								

Week 19:
The BMI (Body Mass Index) Concept

What Is the BMI (Body Mass Index)?

BMI or Body Mass Index is an estimate of total body fat based on your height and weight. It's important to know your BMI because excess body fat can put you at risk for health problems such as cancer, cardiovascular disease, and diabetes. To calculate your BMI yourself, use this formula: (weight in pounds x 703)/height in inches multiplied by itself. Once you've determined your BMI, you can determine whether you're in the underweight, normal weight, overweight or obese category. Here are the guidelines:

- Underweight: BMI of less than 18.5
- Normal Weight: BMI of 18.5-24.9
- Overweight: BMI of 25.0 to 29.9
- Obese: BMI of 30.0 or more

Your doctor or health care provider will take more than BMI into account when evaluating your health—your waist circumference and other lifestyle issues (such as a history of heart disease or your smoking status) may also affect your risk of certain health conditions. For people who are athletes and who have muscular builds, the BMI may overestimate total body fat, since muscle weighs more than fat. And in seniors or those who have lost muscle mass, the BMI may underestimate body fat.

However, because the vast majority—80 percent to 90 percent—of diabetics are overweight or obese when first diagnosed, it is important to get your BMI as low as possible as part of your medically-supervised diabetes management program; remember, don't fall victim to fad diets that are dangerous for diabetics. Instead, develop a balanced, medically-sound program with your diabetes healthcare team.

How Can I Better Manage My BMI?

As shown in several studies, the best way to achieve a healthy BMI and maintain it is to combine a common-sense diet with fewer calories eaten than you burn up each day. For diabetics, this means eating no more than about six hundred calories per meal combined with thirty to forty-five minutes per day of your favorite moderate activity such as walking, gardening, swimming, or biking. There is no need to use extreme diet or exercise programs; *The Paleo Diet* and *The Low-Starch Diabetes Solution* offer programs that allow you to eat regular foods like everyone else with only a few simple requirements, and regular activity is the way you keep the weight from coming back once it is lost.

One way to think about achieving a healthy BMI is "slow and steady as she goes." By adopting a new lifestyle that utilizes *The Paleo Diet* or *The Low-Starch Diabetes Solution* as its foundation, you can enjoy your food, your activity, and most of all—a new and healthier BMI. As long as you continue to burn more calories each day than you consume, you will lose weight and keep it off. Even if you slip a day here and a day there, what really counts is what you do over the course of a full week; as long as your net weekly calories burned exceed those consumed, you will lose weight.

BMI Information Resources

1. American Diabetes Association http://www.diabetes.org/food-and-fitness/fitness/weight-loss/bmi-calculator.html
2. The National Institute of Diabetes and Digestive and Kidney Diseases Weight Control Information Network at http://win.niddk.nih.gov/publications/tools.htm
3. Centers for Disease Control and Prevention (CDC) at http://www.cdc.gov/nccdphp/dnpa/bmi/calc-bmi.htm

Reviewed by: **Jay Krakovitz, M.D.**, for:

DIABETES SELF-DEFENSE, LLC
6360 Quail Street, Denver, CO 80004
Cell: 303-931-9710; **Web:** www.DiabetesSelfDefense.com

Week Beginning: _____

Weekly Record

MON:	Time	Bld Sgr	Meals	Net Carbs(g)	2 Hrs Bld Sgr	Blood Press	Exercise/Min	Notes/Sickness
Breakfast								
Lunch								
Dinner								
Bedtime								

TUES:	Time	Bld Sgr	Meals	Net Carbs(g)	2 Hrs Bld Sgr	Blood Press	Exercise/Min	Notes/Sickness
Breakfast								
Lunch								
Dinner								
Bedtime								

WED:	Time	Bld Sgr	Meals	Net Carbs(g)	2 Hrs Bld Sgr	Blood Press	Exercise/Min	Notes/Sickness
Breakfast								
Lunch								
Dinner								
Bedtime								

THUR:	Time	Bld Sgr	Meals	Net Carbs(g)	2 Hrs Bld Sgr	Blood Press	Exercise/Min	Notes/Sickness
Breakfast								
Lunch								
Dinner								
Bedtime								

FRI:	Time	Bld Sgr	Meals	Net Carbs(g)	2 Hrs Bld Sgr	Blood Press	Exercise/Min	Notes/Sickness
Breakfast								
Lunch								
Dinner								
Bedtime								

SAT:	Time	Bld Sgr	Meals	Net Carbs(g)	2 Hrs Bld Sgr	Blood Press	Exercise/Min	Notes/Sickness
Breakfast								
Lunch								
Dinner								
Bedtime								

SUN:	Time	Bld Sgr	Meals	Net Carbs(g)	2 Hrs Bld Sgr	Blood Press	Exercise/Min	Notes/Sickness
Breakfast								
Lunch								
Dinner								
Bedtime								

Week 20:
Exercise and Diabetes Management

What Does Science Say about Exercise and Diabetes Management?

Regular exercise is supported by many scientific studies and is a recommended component of diabetes management. In both Type 1 and Type 2 diabetes mellitus, regular exercise can help to increase insulin sensitivity, lower blood glucose, reduce blood cholesterol, and have positive psychological effects. More markedly in Type 2 than in Type 1, regular physical activity improves blood sugar control, reduces high blood pressure, and normalizes cholesterol and triglycerides.

Adjustments in insulin dosage, careful blood sugar monitoring, and attention to diet around the time of exercise will help prevent hypoglycemia and hyperglycemia, which are common hazards of exercise in diabetes. Special precautions are necessary for those who have diabetic complications such as retinopathy or peripheral neuropathy; always check with your doctor before beginning any new exercise program.

Why Should I Be Concerned about Exercise?

With regular exercise, overall well-being improves, cardiovascular risk factors are reduced, and high blood sugars are better controlled. The American Diabetes Association (ADA) concludes its position statement on exercise with the injunction that "all patients with diabetes should have the opportunity to benefit from the many valuable effects of exercise." In fact, findings presented at the Sixty-Eighth Annual Scientific Sessions of the ADA in 2008 revealed this: the combined results of several clinical trials suggest that regular exercise has a beneficial overall effect on diabetic subjects, reducing cardiovascular risk and, notably, the risk of stroke.

At the same time, exercise presents risks for some patients, imposing the need for specific activity precautions, careful planning of the timing of physical activity, and realistic limits on the duration and type of activity. The clinical picture differs between Types 1 and 2 diabetes. The former patients often want to exercise but sometimes should not, while the latter almost always should exercise but often don't want to. The exercise prescription must be tailored to the disease, the individual, and his or her fluctuating condition. Be sure to work closely with your diabetes healthcare team on your plan.

How Can I Incorporate Exercise into My Diabetes Management Plan?

When you're ready to exercise, start slowly. Work your way up to thirty minutes of moderate-intensity exercise most days of the week. Here are some good general tips: (1) *Check your blood sugar.* Check your blood sugar before, during and after exercise—especially if you take insulin or medications that can cause low blood sugar (hypoglycemia). Carry glucose tablets or hard candy in case your blood sugar drops too low or you feel shaky, nervous, or confused; (2) *Watch your feet.* Wear comfortable socks and athletic shoes. Check your feet before and after exercise for any signs of potential damage, such as cuts or blisters; (3) *Stay hydrated.* Drink plenty of fluids while you exercise, especially when it's hot. Dehydration can increase your blood sugar. If you exercise for more than an hour, drink carbohydrate-containing beverages rather than plain water; (4) *ID yourself.* Wear a diabetes identification bracelet or shoe tag while exercising in case of an emergency; (5) *Know when to rest or stop.* If you experience any warning signs—severe shortness of breath, dizziness, faintness, nausea, chest pain, heart palpitations, or pain in an arm or in your jaw—stop exercising. If you don't feel better within fifteen minutes, seek immediate medical help. You will need to be your own personal coach when it comes to exercising safely.

Exercise and Diabetes Information Resources

1. The Mayo Clinic at http://www.mayoclinic.com/health/diabetes-and-exercise/DA00105
2. The American Diabetes Association at http://www.diabetes.org/food-and-fitness/fitness/

Reviewed by: **Jay Krakovitz, M.D.,** for:

DIABETES SELF-DEFENSE, LLC
6360 Quail Street, Denver, CO 80004
Cell: 303-931-9710; **Web:** www.DiabetesSelfDefense.com

Week Beginning: _____

Weekly Record

MON:	Time	Bld Sgr	Meals	Net Carbs(g)	2 Hrs Bld Sgr	Blood Press	Exercise/Min	Notes/Sickness
Breakfast								
Lunch								
Dinner								
Bedtime								

TUES:	Time	Bld Sgr	Meals	Net Carbs(g)	2 Hrs Bld Sgr	Blood Press	Exercise/Min	Notes/Sickness
Breakfast								
Lunch								
Dinner								
Bedtime								

WED:	Time	Bld Sgr	Meals	Net Carbs(g)	2 Hrs Bld Sgr	Blood Press	Exercise/Min	Notes/Sickness
Breakfast								
Lunch								
Dinner								
Bedtime								

THUR:	Time	Bld Sgr	Meals	Net Carbs(g)	2 Hrs Bld Sgr	Blood Press	Exercise/Min	Notes/Sickness
Breakfast								
Lunch								
Dinner								
Bedtime								

FRI:	Time	Bld Sgr	Meals	Net Carbs(g)	2 Hrs Bld Sgr	Blood Press	Exercise/Min	Notes/Sickness
Breakfast								
Lunch								
Dinner								
Bedtime								

SAT:	Time	Bld Sgr	Meals	Net Carbs(g)	2 Hrs Bld Sgr	Blood Press	Exercise/Min	Notes/Sickness
Breakfast								
Lunch								
Dinner								
Bedtime								

SUN:	Time	Bld Sgr	Meals	Net Carbs(g)	2 Hrs Bld Sgr	Blood Press	Exercise/Min	Notes/Sickness
Breakfast								
Lunch								
Dinner								
Bedtime								

Week 21:
Comparing the Low-Carb, Mediterranean, and Low-Fat Diets

What Does Science Say about the Various Weight Loss Diets Being Promoted Today?

There have been a lot of weight-loss diets promoted in recent years, from the *Atkins Diet* to the *South Beach Diet* to *Weight Watchers;* most of these diets usually have few to none of their own clinical studies. However, the prestigious *New England Journal of Medicine* conducted a two-year trial for three of the more popular diet programs and published their results in July, 2008, among moderately obese subjects (mean age, 52 years; mean BMI, 31; male sex, 86 percent) to one of three diets: *low-fat*, restricted calorie; *Mediterranean*, restricted-calorie; or *low-carbohydrate*, non-restricted calorie. The study concluded that the Low-Carb and Mediterranean diets are effective alternatives to low-fat diets, and in fact, had more favorable effects on weight, blood fats (low-carb), and glycemic control (Mediterranean) than the low-fat approach.

Why Should I Be Concerned about the Results of a Diet Comparison Test?

Among the 272 participants who completed the test, thirty-six had diabetes. The two areas of control that were more favorable among people with diabetes on the Mediterranean diet vs. the low-fat diet were:

- Fasting Plasma Glucose;
- Insulin Levels

In summary, then, it would appear that the Low-Carb and Mediterranean Diets may offer superior diabetes control versus traditional Low-Fat diets. The authors of the study also recommend that individual preferences and individual metabolism levels need to be considered when selecting the best dietary approach.

Diabetes and Diet Information Resources

1. Shai, Iris, et al, "Weight Loss with a Low-Carb, Mediterranean, or Low-Fat Diet," *The New England Journal of Medicine*, July 17, 2008, Number 3, Volume 359:229-241.

Reviewed by: **Jay Krakovitz, M.D.,** for:

DIABETES SELF-DEFENSE, LLC
6360 Quail Street, Denver, CO 80004
Cell: 303-931-9710; **Web:** www.DiabetesSelfDefense.com

Week Beginning: _____

Weekly Record

MON:	Time	Bld Sgr	Meals	Net Carbs(g)	2 Hrs Bld Sgr	Blood Press	Exercise/Min	Notes/Sickness
Breakfast								
Lunch								
Dinner								
Bedtime								

TUES:	Time	Bld Sgr	Meals	Net Carbs(g)	2 Hrs Bld Sgr	Blood Press	Exercise/Min	Notes/Sickness
Breakfast								
Lunch								
Dinner								
Bedtime								

WED:	Time	Bld Sgr	Meals	Net Carbs(g)	2 Hrs Bld Sgr	Blood Press	Exercise/Min	Notes/Sickness
Breakfast								
Lunch								
Dinner								
Bedtime								

THUR:	Time	Bld Sgr	Meals	Net Carbs(g)	2 Hrs Bld Sgr	Blood Press	Exercise/Min	Notes/Sickness
Breakfast								
Lunch								
Dinner								
Bedtime								

FRI:	Time	Bld Sgr	Meals	Net Carbs(g)	2 Hrs Bld Sgr	Blood Press	Exercise/Min	Notes/Sickness
Breakfast								
Lunch								
Dinner								
Bedtime								

SAT:	Time	Bld Sgr	Meals	Net Carbs(g)	2 Hrs Bld Sgr	Blood Press	Exercise/Min	Notes/Sickness
Breakfast								
Lunch								
Dinner								
Bedtime								

SUN:	Time	Bld Sgr	Meals	Net Carbs(g)	2 Hrs Bld Sgr	Blood Press	Exercise/Min	Notes/Sickness
Breakfast								
Lunch								
Dinner								
Bedtime								

Week 22:
Diabetes Medications That Can Help

What Does Science Say About Byetta® (Exenatide) and Symlin® (Pramlintide)?

Exenatide (brand name *Byetta®*) is the first in a new class of drugs for the treatment of type 2 diabetes called incretin mimetics. Exenatide is a synthetic version of exendin-4, a naturally-occurring hormone that was first isolated from the saliva of the lizard known as a Gila monster. Exenatide works to lower blood glucose levels primarily by increasing insulin secretion. Because it only has this effect in the presence of elevated blood glucose levels, it does not tend to increase the risk of hypoglycemia on its own, although hypoglycemia can occur if taken in conjunction with a sulfonylurea. The primary side effect is nausea, which tends to improve over time.

Pramlintide (brand name *Symlin®*) is a synthetic form of the hormone amylin, which is produced along with insulin by the beta cells in the pancreas. Amylin, insulin, and another hormone, glucagon, work in an interrelated fashion to maintain normal blood glucose levels.

Because of differences in chemistry, pramlintide cannot be combined in the same vial or syringe with insulin and must be injected separately. Pramlintide has been approved for people with Type 1 diabetes who are not achieving their goal A1C levels and for people with Type 2 diabetes who are using insulin and are not achieving their A1C goals.

Why Should I Be Interested in Byetta and Symlin?

Byetta® is injected with meals, and patients using Byetta® have generally experienced modest weight loss as well as improved glycemic control. Byetta® has been approved for use by people with Type 2 diabetes who have not achieved their target A1C levels using metformin, a sulfonylurea, or a combination of metformin and a sulfonylurea.

Symlin® injections taken with meals have been shown to modestly improve A1C levels without causing increased hypoglycemia or weight gain, and Symlin even promotes modest weight loss. The primary side effect is nausea, which tends to improve over time and as an individual patient determines his or her optimal dose.

How Can Byetta or Symlin Be Used in My Diabetes Management Program?

Talk to your doctor About whether or not Byetta® or Symlin® make sense for you and your personal diabetes management program. David Mendosa, a well-known diabetes writer on the web, has experienced great success with Byetta and also written a book about it, *Losing Weight with Your Diabetes Medication.*

Byetta® and Symlin® Information Resources

1. The American Diabetes Association, "Other Diabetes Medications," at http://www.diabetes.org/type-2-diabetes/oral-medications.jsp
2. Mendosa, David, "Losing Weight With Your Diabetes Medication: How Byetta and Other Drugs Can Help You Lose More Weight Than You Ever Thought Possible," (Marlowe Diabetes Library). © 2007, at http://www.amazon.com/Losing-Weight-Diabetes-Medication-ebook/dp/B0042JSNL8/ref=sr_1_1?s=digital-text Andie=UTF8 Andqid=1309558098 Andsr=1-1

Part 5:
"R" = Regular Medical Management

"R" Section Summary

If a healthy diet is the foundation of an effective diabetes management program, then Regular Medical Management is the first floor. For those with Type 1 diabetes, insulin means the difference between life or death. For those with Type 2 diabetes, regular medical management means the difference between controlling or not controlling their diabetes. Because diabetes is a twenty-four-seven disease, you have to be a twenty-four-seven watchdog, keeping daily tabs on your diet, medications, and blood sugar with weekly and quarterly checks of your blood pressure, cholesterol, and weight. While you must be the "quarterback" or leader of your diabetes healthcare team, you also need to be open to advice from your "coaches": your primary care physician, your nutritionist, your dentist, your eye doctor, and any other medical specialists you are referred to.

Reviewed by: **Jay Krakovitz, M.D.,** for:

DIABETES SELF-DEFENSE, LLC
6360 Quail Street, Denver, CO 80004
Cell: 303-931-9710; **Web:** www.DiabetesSelfDefense.com

Week Beginning: _____

Weekly Record

MON:	Time	Bld Sgr	Meals	Net Carbs(g)	2 Hrs Bld Sgr	Blood Press	Exercise/Min	Notes/Sickness
Breakfast								
Lunch								
Dinner								
Bedtime								

TUES:	Time	Bld Sgr	Meals	Net Carbs(g)	2 Hrs Bld Sgr	Blood Press	Exercise/Min	Notes/Sickness
Breakfast								
Lunch								
Dinner								
Bedtime								

WED:	Time	Bld Sgr	Meals	Net Carbs(g)	2 Hrs Bld Sgr	Blood Press	Exercise/Min	Notes/Sickness
Breakfast								
Lunch								
Dinner								
Bedtime								

THUR:	Time	Bld Sgr	Meals	Net Carbs(g)	2 Hrs Bld Sgr	Blood Press	Exercise/Min	Notes/Sickness
Breakfast								
Lunch								
Dinner								
Bedtime								

FRI:	Time	Bld Sgr	Meals	Net Carbs(g)	2 Hrs Bld Sgr	Blood Press	Exercise/Min	Notes/Sickness
Breakfast								
Lunch								
Dinner								
Bedtime								

SAT:	Time	Bld Sgr	Meals	Net Carbs(g)	2 Hrs Bld Sgr	Blood Press	Exercise/Min	Notes/Sickness
Breakfast								
Lunch								
Dinner								
Bedtime								

SUN:	Time	Bld Sgr	Meals	Net Carbs(g)	2 Hrs Bld Sgr	Blood Press	Exercise/Min	Notes/Sickness
Breakfast								
Lunch								
Dinner								
Bedtime								

Week 23:
The Role of Self-Care in Diabetes

What Does Science Say about the Role of Self-Care in Diabetes?

When people with diabetes are trained in self-care of diabetes, several studies have shown that these individuals gain significantly better diabetes control versus those who are not educated. Self-care of diabetes is especially critical in that, unlike other major diseases such as heart disease and cancer, with diabetes the patient is the one that actually self-administers their medical therapy: measuring their foods and eating properly at the right times, measuring and taking medications properly, and measuring their blood sugar and blood pressure on a regular basis.

Why Should I Be Concerned about Diabetes Self-Care?

The main reason to worry is that if you do not take control of your diabetes through self-management, no one will; moreover, if you do not have your diabetes in good control by personally taking care of it, over time you may experience long-term complications like heart disease, stroke, amputations, and blindness. Without proper self-management and monitoring, you may experience *acute complications* from high blood sugar in the short-run like *diabetic ketoacidosis or HHNS* (Hyperglycemic Hyperosmolar Nonketotic Syndrome) that can result in diabetic coma or death. With diabetes, you have to know what's going on with your body better than anyone else at all times. In other words, you really do need to become "your own best doctor" to help yourself avoid the serious health problems that diabetes can send your way.

How Can I Do a Better Job of Diabetes Self-Care?

To use a football analogy, it's somewhat like you are the *quarterback* of your diabetes healthcare team and your doctor is the coach. Your coach will prepare you for what needs to be done, but you're the one that needs to lead the team. Other diabetes healthcare professionals like your dietitian, eye doctor, kidney specialist, foot doctor, and Certified Diabetes Educator (CDE) all play vital roles on the team and will provide you with feedback and direction). To find a diabetes educator near you, visit the American Association of Diabetes Educators at their website, www.diabeteseducator.org. As the quarterback of the team, you need a solid strategy for managing your diabetes, and the *HEARTS Strategy* is one way to minimize your risk of developing complications:

- *H* = Halt or minimize vices (smoking, caffeine, and junk foods)
- *E* = Eat and drink a healthy diet (high-fiber, low-carb, non-starchy fruits and vegetables)
- *A* = Achieve common sense weight loss and fitness goals (getting more active)
- *R* = Regular medical management (regular check-ups, annual flu shot, records)
- *T* = Targeted nutritional support (dietary supplements, special foods)
- *S* = Study diabetes (get to know diabetes, reading articles, blogs, books, latest research)

Diabetes Self-Care Information Resources

1. Diabetes Self-Management Magazine (www.diabetesselfmanagement.com)
2. The American Association of Diabetes Educators (www.diabeteseducator.org)
3. The National Diabetes Education Program at (www.ndep.nih.gov)

Reviewed by: **Jay Krakovitz, M.D.,** for:

DIABETES SELF-DEFENSE, LLC
6360 Quail Street, Denver, CO 80004
Cell: 303-931-9710; **Web:** www.DiabetesSelfDefense.com

Week Beginning: _____

Weekly Record

MON:	Time	Bld Sgr	Meals	Net Carbs(g)	2 Hrs Bld Sgr	Blood Press	Exercise/Min	Notes/Sickness
Breakfast								
Lunch								
Dinner								
Bedtime								

TUES:	Time	Bld Sgr	Meals	Net Carbs(g)	2 Hrs Bld Sgr	Blood Press	Exercise/Min	Notes/Sickness
Breakfast								
Lunch								
Dinner								
Bedtime								

WED:	Time	Bld Sgr	Meals	Net Carbs(g)	2 Hrs Bld Sgr	Blood Press	Exercise/Min	Notes/Sickness
Breakfast								
Lunch								
Dinner								
Bedtime								

THUR:	Time	Bld Sgr	Meals	Net Carbs(g)	2 Hrs Bld Sgr	Blood Press	Exercise/Min	Notes/Sickness
Breakfast								
Lunch								
Dinner								
Bedtime								

FRI:	Time	Bld Sgr	Meals	Net Carbs(g)	2 Hrs Bld Sgr	Blood Press	Exercise/Min	Notes/Sickness
Breakfast								
Lunch								
Dinner								
Bedtime								

SAT:	Time	Bld Sgr	Meals	Net Carbs(g)	2 Hrs Bld Sgr	Blood Press	Exercise/Min	Notes/Sickness
Breakfast								
Lunch								
Dinner								
Bedtime								

SUN:	Time	Bld Sgr	Meals	Net Carbs(g)	2 Hrs Bld Sgr	Blood Press	Exercise/Min	Notes/Sickness
Breakfast								
Lunch								
Dinner								
Bedtime								

Week 24:
Monitoring the ABCs of Diabetes

What Does Science Say about Managing the ABCs of Diabetes?

Tight management of the ABCs of diabetes, or your A1C (blood glucose or sugar), Blood pressure, and Cholesterol, has been scientifically shown to help reduce the risks of cardiovascular disease, including heart attack, stroke or other diabetes complications. These are called the ABCs of diabetes by the American Diabetes Association (ADA) and the American College of Cardiology (ACC):

- A is for the *A1C test:* It shows how well your blood glucose has been controlled over the last 2-3 months. It should be checked at least twice a year. The goal for most people is less than 7 percent. High blood glucose levels can harm your kidneys, feet, and eyes.
- B is for *Blood Pressure:* The goal for people with diabetes is 130/80 or less. High blood pressure makes your heart work too hard. It can cause heart attack, stroke, and kidney disease.
- C is for *Cholesterol:* The LDL goal for most people with diabetes is less than 100 mg/dL. Bad cholesterol, or LDL, can build up and clog your blood vessels. It can cause a heart attack or a stroke.

Why Should I Be Concerned about the ABCs of Diabetes?

People with diabetes and their doctors are failing to give cholesterol and blood pressure control the attention needed to reduce the high risk for heart attacks and strokes in diabetes, according to four reports in June 2004 at the American Diabetes Association's Sixty-Fourth Annual Scientific Sessions.

Diabetes management requires equal attention to control of blood glucose, cholesterol, blood pressure and other cardiovascular risk factors—but it's not happening, as today's research reports show. Physicians around the world and their patients are failing to make the link science has long since proven—that two out of three people with diabetes die from heart disease and stroke.

—Eugene J. Barrett, MD, PhD,
President of the American Diabetes Association

How Can I Better Control the ABCs of Diabetes?

The tight management of blood glucose (sugar) has long been a cornerstone of diabetes care. Yet research has shown that other cardiovascular risk factors, such as blood pressure and cholesterol, must also be addressed in order to reduce heart attacks and stroke in patients with diabetes. Furthermore, a 2004 study published in the *Journal of the American Medical Association* revealed *less than 8 percent* of people with diabetes meet their appropriate target blood sugar, blood pressure and cholesterol levels; more recent data shows numbers close to 15 percent. The ADA and ACC recently launched an aggressive education initiative called "Make the Link! Diabetes, Heart Disease and Stroke" to illustrate the critical link between diabetes and heart disease, as well as emphasize the importance of comprehensive diabetes management. Your own *unique* diabetes management program of a healthy diet, achieving a healthy weight, regular exercise, and medication, developed with your diabetes healthcare team, can help you gain better control of the ABCs of diabetes. One of the largest and most recent clinical trials, the ACCORD Trial (Action to Control Cardiovascular Risk in Diabetes), which was published in the *New England Journal of Medicine* 2008, revealed that intensive blood sugar control did not significantly reduce cardiovascular events; however, physicians commenting on the study nonetheless still advise that each patient situation is unique and that in many cases "near-normal" blood sugar control may be helpful.

The ABCs of Diabetes" Information Resources

1. The National Diabetes Education Program at http://ndep.nih.gov/diabetes/control/control.htm
2. The American Diabetes Association at http://www.diabetes.org/living-with-diabetes/complications/mens-health/serious-health-implications/abcs-of-heart-disease.html

Week Beginning: _____

Weekly Record

MON:	Time	Bld Sgr	Meals	Net Carbs(g)	2 Hrs Bld Sgr	Blood Press	Exercise/Min	Notes/Sickness
Breakfast								
Lunch								
Dinner								
Bedtime								

TUES:	Time	Bld Sgr	Meals	Net Carbs(g)	2 Hrs Bld Sgr	Blood Press	Exercise/Min	Notes/Sickness
Breakfast								
Lunch								
Dinner								
Bedtime								

WED:	Time	Bld Sgr	Meals	Net Carbs(g)	2 Hrs Bld Sgr	Blood Press	Exercise/Min	Notes/Sickness
Breakfast								
Lunch								
Dinner								
Bedtime								

THUR:	Time	Bld Sgr	Meals	Net Carbs(g)	2 Hrs Bld Sgr	Blood Press	Exercise/Min	Notes/Sickness
Breakfast								
Lunch								
Dinner								
Bedtime								

FRI:	Time	Bld Sgr	Meals	Net Carbs(g)	2 Hrs Bld Sgr	Blood Press	Exercise/Min	Notes/Sickness
Breakfast								
Lunch								
Dinner								
Bedtime								

SAT:	Time	Bld Sgr	Meals	Net Carbs(g)	2 Hrs Bld Sgr	Blood Press	Exercise/Min	Notes/Sickness
Breakfast								
Lunch								
Dinner								
Bedtime								

SUN:	Time	Bld Sgr	Meals	Net Carbs(g)	2 Hrs Bld Sgr	Blood Press	Exercise/Min	Notes/Sickness
Breakfast								
Lunch								
Dinner								
Bedtime								

Week 25:
Intensive Control: ACCORD Pros and Cons

What Does Science Say about the Importance of "Tight" Blood Sugar Control—Keeping Blood Sugar as Close to Normal as Possible (80-120 mg/dL)?

Five-year results of the Action to Control Cardiovascular Risk in Diabetes (ACCORD) study confirm that neither more intensive lowering of blood glucose (sugar) levels, more intensive lowering of blood pressure, nor treatment of blood lipids with a fibrate and a statin drug reduce cardiovascular risk in people with established Type 2 diabetes who are at severely high risk for cardiovascular events. However, the study did find improvements to microvascular conditions, such as progression of diabetic eye disease (retinopathy), visual acuity, and renal and nerve function. The landmark study is sponsored by the federal government through the National Institutes of Health (NIH).

Speaking at the American Diabetes Association's seventieth Scientific Sessions, the ACCORD Study Group cautioned that any potential benefits must be weighed against the increased risk of mortality and episodes of seriously low blood glucose that were seen to accompany intensive lowering of blood glucose levels—which in ACCORD was focused on achieving normal A1C levels in the study population. They emphasized that both the positive and negative results of the study apply only to this population of middle-aged or older people with Type 2 diabetes for an average of ten years who also had a history of cardiovascular disease (CVD) or at least two risk factors for CVD.

What Does the American Diabetes Association Say about These Findings?

In response to the announcement by the National Heart, Lung, and Blood Institute, which sponsored the ACCORD (Action to Control Cardiovascular Risk in Diabetes) Trial, the American Diabetes Association strongly encourages people with diabetes not to alter their course of treatment without first consulting with their health care team. The American Diabetes Association continues to encourage good control of blood glucose, blood pressure, and cholesterol for the individualized management of diabetes and its complications.

How Should I Use the Latest Findings on Tight Blood Sugar Control?

The American Diabetes Association's 2011 Standards of Medical Care state that blood sugar treatment should be tailored to the individual patient and that for some people with diabetes, intensive blood sugar control may not be warranted. Of note, the American Diabetes Association (in its Standards of Medical Care) states:

> Less stringent A1C goals may be appropriate for patients with a history of severe hypoglycemia, patients with limited life expectancies, children, individuals with comorbid conditions, and those with longstanding diabetes and minimal or stable microvascular complications.

In short, work closely with your doctor and your diabetes healthcare team to develop the best program for your unique situation.

"Tight" or Intensive Blood Sugar Control Information Resources

1. The American Diabetes Association http://www.diabetes.org/for-media/2008/statement-from-the-american.html?utm_source=WWW Andutm_medium=GSA Andutm_content=keymatch-ACCORD Andutm_campaign=PR
2. *Medical News Today*, "Mixed Results From ACCORD: Study Found No Overall Reduction In Cardiovascular Risk, But Benefits To Eyes, Kidneys and Nerves," http://www.medicalnewstoday.com/printerfriendlynews.php?newsid=193313

Reviewed by: **Jay Krakovitz, M.D.,** for:

DIABETES SELF-DEFENSE, LLC
6360 Quail Street, Denver, CO 80004
Cell: 303-931-9710; **Web:** www.DiabetesSelfDefense.com

Week Beginning: _____

Weekly Record

MON:	Time	Bld Sgr	Meals	Net Carbs(g)	2 Hrs Bld Sgr	Blood Press	Exercise/Min	Notes/Sickness
Breakfast								
Lunch								
Dinner								
Bedtime								

TUES:	Time	Bld Sgr	Meals	Net Carbs(g)	2 Hrs Bld Sgr	Blood Press	Exercise/Min	Notes/Sickness
Breakfast								
Lunch								
Dinner								
Bedtime								

WED:	Time	Bld Sgr	Meals	Net Carbs(g)	2 Hrs Bld Sgr	Blood Press	Exercise/Min	Notes/Sickness
Breakfast								
Lunch								
Dinner								
Bedtime								

THUR:	Time	Bld Sgr	Meals	Net Carbs(g)	2 Hrs Bld Sgr	Blood Press	Exercise/Min	Notes/Sickness
Breakfast								
Lunch								
Dinner								
Bedtime								

FRI:	Time	Bld Sgr	Meals	Net Carbs(g)	2 Hrs Bld Sgr	Blood Press	Exercise/Min	Notes/Sickness
Breakfast								
Lunch								
Dinner								
Bedtime								

SAT:	Time	Bld Sgr	Meals	Net Carbs(g)	2 Hrs Bld Sgr	Blood Press	Exercise/Min	Notes/Sickness
Breakfast								
Lunch								
Dinner								
Bedtime								

SUN:	Time	Bld Sgr	Meals	Net Carbs(g)	2 Hrs Bld Sgr	Blood Press	Exercise/Min	Notes/Sickness
Breakfast								
Lunch								
Dinner								
Bedtime								

Week 26:
Diabetes and High Blood Pressure

What Does Science Say about Diabetes and High Blood Pressure?

High blood pressure or hypertension must be a primary health concern for people with diabetes. Up to 73 percent of diabetics are estimated to have high blood pressure. Blood pressure refers to the pressure required for the heart to pump blood through the arteries to all parts of the body. Blood pressure is defined as the force in the arteries when the heart beats (systolic pressure) and when the heart is at rest (diastolic pressure), and it's measured in millimeters of mercury (mm Hg). When a person with diabetes has high blood pressure that means additional pressure is needed to get blood to and from the heart, possibly indicating a blood vessel blockage of some sort like cholesterol or a thickening of the blood vessel linings.

Why Should I Worry about High Blood Pressure?

First of all, people with diabetes are at higher than normal risk than the general population for serious diseases related to blood vessel complications, including heart disease, kidney failure, blindness, and nerve disorders. High blood pressure can not only make these conditions worse, it is also the leading risk factor for stroke. High blood pressure must be treated aggressively in all patients with diabetes, yet recent studies show that this is not being done enough. Make sure you talk to your doctor about measuring and treating your blood pressure. In their national program to fight diabetes, the American Diabetes Association advises diabetics to "Know The ABCs of Diabetes," where the *B* stands for *blood pressure*. It's that important.

How Can I Control High Blood Pressure?

Normalizing blood pressure will help prevent damage to your eyes, kidneys, heart, and blood vessels. Blood pressure is written with two numbers divided by a slash. For example: 120/70. The first number should be 130 or below, and the second number should be 80 or below. Your goal is to keep your blood pressure at 130/80 or below. If your blood pressure is too high, your doctor may ask you to take a blood pressure medicine called an *ARB* (angiotensin II receptor blocker) like Cozaar® or an ACE (angiotensin converting enzyme) inhibitor like Altace®.

It is also important, unless you are on a potassium-restricted diet for medical reasons, to increase the ratio of potassium-rich foods such as whole-grains, fruits, vegetables, and nuts in your diet relative to the amount of sodium you consume, striving to achieve a ratio of *3:1* or higher; the National Institute of Medicine now recommends consuming 4700 mg of potassium and 1500 mg of sodium each day.

Make sure you carefully read food labels on all packaged foods, especially the so-called health foods. Finally, achieving a healthy weight, regular exercise, limiting alcohol, and controlling stress have also been shown to reduce blood pressure significantly; the *Journal of Hypertension* in January, 2005 revealed that only sixty to ninety minutes of exercise per week was enough to significantly lower blood pressure. Of course, it is strongly recommended that any diabetic also quit smoking not only because of the increased lung cancer risk, but also because of the increased risk of high blood pressure. In fact, in 2012 results from the *Copenhagen City Heart Study* revealed that jogging one to one and a half hours per week could extend one's life expectancy by six years.

Diabetes and High Blood Pressure Information Resources

1. The American Diabetes Association Position Statement: "Hypertension Management in Adults With Diabetes," http://care.diabetesjournals.org/cgi/reprint/27/suppl_1/s65
2. Hypertension and diabetes at http://www.ncbi.nlm.nih.gov/pubmed/18230957

Reviewed by: **Jay Krakovitz, M.D.,** for:

DIABETES SELF-DEFENSE, LLC
6360 Quail Street, Denver, CO 80004
Cell: 303-931-9710; **Web:** www.DiabetesSelfDefense.com

Week Beginning: _____

Weekly Record

MON:	Time	Bld Sgr	Meals	Net Carbs(g)	2 Hrs Bld Sgr	Blood Press	Exercise/Min	Notes/Sickness
Breakfast								
Lunch								
Dinner								
Bedtime								

TUES:	Time	Bld Sgr	Meals	Net Carbs(g)	2 Hrs Bld Sgr	Blood Press	Exercise/Min	Notes/Sickness
Breakfast								
Lunch								
Dinner								
Bedtime								

WED:	Time	Bld Sgr	Meals	Net Carbs(g)	2 Hrs Bld Sgr	Blood Press	Exercise/Min	Notes/Sickness
Breakfast								
Lunch								
Dinner								
Bedtime								

THUR:	Time	Bld Sgr	Meals	Net Carbs(g)	2 Hrs Bld Sgr	Blood Press	Exercise/Min	Notes/Sickness
Breakfast								
Lunch								
Dinner								
Bedtime								

FRI:	Time	Bld Sgr	Meals	Net Carbs(g)	2 Hrs Bld Sgr	Blood Press	Exercise/Min	Notes/Sickness
Breakfast								
Lunch								
Dinner								
Bedtime								

SAT:	Time	Bld Sgr	Meals	Net Carbs(g)	2 Hrs Bld Sgr	Blood Press	Exercise/Min	Notes/Sickness
Breakfast								
Lunch								
Dinner								
Bedtime								

SUN:	Time	Bld Sgr	Meals	Net Carbs(g)	2 Hrs Bld Sgr	Blood Press	Exercise/Min	Notes/Sickness
Breakfast								
Lunch								
Dinner								
Bedtime								

Week 27:
Diabetes and Blood Fats

What Does Science Say about Diabetes and Blood Fats (Cholesterol and Triglycerides)?

Cholesterol is a normally found in the body in cell walls and membranes, vitamin D, hormones, and fat-digesting enzymes. Excess cholesterol can get deposited in the walls of blood vessels, leading to *atherosclerosis*, or hardening of the arteries. Atherosclerosis leads to heart attack and stroke. Cholesterol is divided into HDL and LDL (bad cholesterol), which carries cholesterol in the blood and can get deposited onto the walls of blood vessels, causing atherosclerotic plaques. HDL (good cholesterol) helps clear the blood of cholesterol, and may even remove cholesterol from atherosclerotic blood vessels. *Triglycerides* are a type of fat found in the bloodstream and in fat tissue. High levels of triglycerides contribute to atherosclerosis. Very high levels of triglycerides can cause pancreatitis (inflammation of the pancreas).

Managing cholesterol is such a critical issue for diabetics that the American Diabetes Association has labeled it the "C" component of their *Know Your ABCs of Diabetes* national campaign. High blood cholesterol/triglycerides are part of the metabolic syndrome, a precursor of diabetes, along with high blood sugar, high blood pressure, and obesity. Up to 80 percent of diabetics are estimated to have high blood cholesterol. The American Diabetes Association and the National Diabetes Education Program recommend that people with diabetes lower their low-density lipoprotein (LDL, or bad cholesterol) levels to 100 mg/dL or below; the goal for triglycerides is 150 mg/dL or below.

Why Should I Worry about High Cholesterol/Triglycerides?

People with diabetes are at higher than normal risk than the general population for serious diseases related to blood vessel complications, including heart disease, kidney failure, blindness, and nerve disorders. High blood cholesterol can not only make these conditions worse, it is also a risk factor for stroke. High blood cholesterol and high triglycerides must be treated aggressively in all patients with diabetes, yet recent studies show that this is not being done enough. Make sure you talk to your doctor about measuring and aggressively treating your high cholesterol with diet, medications, and exercise.

How Can I Control High Cholesterol/Triglycerides?

Keeping your blood cholesterol and triglycerides in the recommended ranges will help prevent damage to your heart, kidneys, and blood vessels. Your doctor will try to help you obtain normal levels of cholesterol and triglycerides through a high-fiber diet, achieving a modest weight loss if overweight, daily exercise, and prescribed medications like statins (Lipitor®, Zocor®). Recently, the April 2004 issue of the *Annals of Internal Medicine* published clinical guidelines stating that nearly all people who have Type 2 diabetes could benefit from treatment with moderate doses of statins because of the effectiveness of these drugs in reducing the risk of developing heart disease. While aging and family history have some influence on your cholesterol levels, the recommended dietary and lifestyle changes along with statins represent the greatest cholesterol-lowering opportunity for people with diabetes.

High Blood Cholesterol and Diabetes Information Resources

1. "Lipid Control in the Management of Type 2 Diabetes Mellitus," *Annals of Internal Medicine* 2004 Apr 20; 140(8):644-9.
2. Behall, K. *American Journal of Clinical Nutrition*, November 2004; vol 80: pp 1185-1193. National Cholesterol Education Program, "*High Blood Cholesterol: What You Need to Know.*"
3. Kowalski, Robert E., "The New 8 Week Cholesterol Cure," © 2002, HarperCollins Books

Reviewed by: **Jay Krakovitz, M.D.,** for:

DIABETES SELF-DEFENSE, LLC
6360 Quail Street, Denver, CO 80004
Cell: 303-931-9710; **Web:** www.DiabetesSelfDefense.com

Week Beginning: _____

Weekly Record

MON:	Time	Bld Sgr	Meals	Net Carbs(g)	2 Hrs Bld Sgr	Blood Press	Exercise/Min	Notes/Sickness
Breakfast								
Lunch								
Dinner								
Bedtime								

TUES:	Time	Bld Sgr	Meals	Net Carbs(g)	2 Hrs Bld Sgr	Blood Press	Exercise/Min	Notes/Sickness
Breakfast								
Lunch								
Dinner								
Bedtime								

WED:	Time	Bld Sgr	Meals	Net Carbs(g)	2 Hrs Bld Sgr	Blood Press	Exercise/Min	Notes/Sickness
Breakfast								
Lunch								
Dinner								
Bedtime								

THUR:	Time	Bld Sgr	Meals	Net Carbs(g)	2 Hrs Bld Sgr	Blood Press	Exercise/Min	Notes/Sickness
Breakfast								
Lunch								
Dinner								
Bedtime								

FRI:	Time	Bld Sgr	Meals	Net Carbs(g)	2 Hrs Bld Sgr	Blood Press	Exercise/Min	Notes/Sickness
Breakfast								
Lunch								
Dinner								
Bedtime								

SAT:	Time	Bld Sgr	Meals	Net Carbs(g)	2 Hrs Bld Sgr	Blood Press	Exercise/Min	Notes/Sickness
Breakfast								
Lunch								
Dinner								
Bedtime								

SUN:	Time	Bld Sgr	Meals	Net Carbs(g)	2 Hrs Bld Sgr	Blood Press	Exercise/Min	Notes/Sickness
Breakfast								
Lunch								
Dinner								
Bedtime								

Week 28:
Medical and Dental Diabetes Examinations

What Does Science Say about Regular Medical and Dental Exams for People with Diabetes?

Studies have shown that those people with diabetes or pre-diabetes that have regular medical and dental examinations are better able to prevent and/or minimize the long-term complications of diabetes such as heart disease, stroke, kidney failure, blindness, and amputations. A diabetes medical/dental checklist can be found in the Appendix.

Why Should I Worry about Regular Medical and Dental Examinations?

Having diabetes places you at a substantially higher risk of major health problems and premature death than the general population. Having uncontrolled diabetes means you have, versus the non-diabetic population: *two to four times* the risk of heart attack; *two to four times* the risk of stroke; *ten times* the risk of blindness; *ten times* the risk of kidney failure; and *three times* the risk of cancer. However, with regular medical and dental exams, you can help minimize the risk of these problems with professional medical guidance and treatment. While there are no guarantees in life or in diabetes, the evidence is in: by having regular exams and taking proper medication and with nutritional and lifestyle changes, you can ward off or minimize the occurrence of these serious health issues of diabetes.

How Should I Prepare for Medical and Dental Examinations?

The key to being a great patient is great preparation. Whether you are having your regular quarterly exam with your regular doctor or are going to a new doctor for the first time, make sure you have the following items checked off your list before your visit:

- Your most current health records for the past two to three months. Ideally, these records will include your weight, blood sugar, blood pressure, and cholesterol levels along with your personal notes as to any physical problems or illnesses: cuts, bruises, flu, fever, etc.
- All important medical/dental insurance information and your insurance card; call your insurance company ahead of time if you're unsure as to what is covered and what isn't. If you are on Medicare or Medicaid, be sure to bring your ID card.
- Method of payment; call the doctor's office ahead of your appointment to see what forms of payment are preferred for your payment or co-pay: credit card, check, etc.

Diabetes and Medical Examination Information Resources

1. The American Diabetes Association Position Statement: Standards of Medical Care In Diabetes, *Diabetes Care* 31: (1) S12, 2008.
2. Clinical Guidelines for Adults With Diabetes, Joslin Diabetes Center and Joslin Clinic at 617-732-2400.
3. Diabetes For Dummies at http://www.dummies.com/how-to/content/diabetes-for-dummies-cheat-sheet.html

Reviewed by: **Jay Krakovitz, M.D.,** for:

DIABETES SELF-DEFENSE, LLC
6360 Quail Street, Denver, CO 80004
Cell: 303-931-9710; **Web:** www.DiabetesSelfDefense.com

Week Beginning: _____

Weekly Record

MON:	Time	Bld Sgr	Meals	Net Carbs(g)	2 Hrs Bld Sgr	Blood Press	Exercise/Min	Notes/Sickness
Breakfast								
Lunch								
Dinner								
Bedtime								

TUES:	Time	Bld Sgr	Meals	Net Carbs(g)	2 Hrs Bld Sgr	Blood Press	Exercise/Min	Notes/Sickness
Breakfast								
Lunch								
Dinner								
Bedtime								

WED:	Time	Bld Sgr	Meals	Net Carbs(g)	2 Hrs Bld Sgr	Blood Press	Exercise/Min	Notes/Sickness
Breakfast								
Lunch								
Dinner								
Bedtime								

THUR:	Time	Bld Sgr	Meals	Net Carbs(g)	2 Hrs Bld Sgr	Blood Press	Exercise/Min	Notes/Sickness
Breakfast								
Lunch								
Dinner								
Bedtime								

FRI:	Time	Bld Sgr	Meals	Net Carbs(g)	2 Hrs Bld Sgr	Blood Press	Exercise/Min	Notes/Sickness
Breakfast								
Lunch								
Dinner								
Bedtime								

SAT:	Time	Bld Sgr	Meals	Net Carbs(g)	2 Hrs Bld Sgr	Blood Press	Exercise/Min	Notes/Sickness
Breakfast								
Lunch								
Dinner								
Bedtime								

SUN:	Time	Bld Sgr	Meals	Net Carbs(g)	2 Hrs Bld Sgr	Blood Press	Exercise/Min	Notes/Sickness
Breakfast								
Lunch								
Dinner								
Bedtime								

Week 29:
High and Low Blood Sugar Emergencies

What Does Science Say about Managing High and Low Blood Sugars?

Medical emergencies can arise for the diabetic patient when their blood sugar is too high (hyperglycemia) or too low (hypoglycemia) for any significant period of time, even a period of time as short as 1 hour. Very high blood sugar is traditionally defined as 250 mg/dL or higher, and low blood sugar or hypoglycemia is defined as 60 mg/dL or lower; normal blood sugar is considered to be 80-120 mg/dL.

In general, people with diabetes that use insulin are most vulnerable to blood sugar that's either too high or too low, but certain oral diabetes medications like sulfonylureas can cause hypoglycemia. Blood sugars that are too high or too low can be equally damaging and dangerous to the body, and even though diabetes is essentially a disease of high blood sugar that needs to be normalized, there is nothing healthy about low blood sugars. High and low blood sugar emergencies occur in people with Type 1, Type 2, and gestational diabetes.

Why Should I Worry about High and Low Blood Sugars?

Failing to properly address either condition quickly can result in severe complications, including kidney failure, diabetic coma, or death. Typical symptoms of hyperglycemia include an intense thirst, a need to urinate frequently, and/or extreme sleepiness or drowsiness, sometimes including blurry vision; if so, drink plenty of water and contact your doctor. Traditional symptoms of low blood sugar include heavy sweating, shakiness, light-headedness, or confusion. Take 15g of fast-acting carbohydrate like glucose tablets or fruit juice, wait ten to fifteen minutes, and test your blood sugar again. Many people, especially the elderly, can suffer from hypoglycemia unawareness, which means they do not feel any symptoms of low blood sugar until they black out or go into diabetic coma.

This is one clear reason why all people with diabetes should always wear an emergency necklace such as a Medic-Alert bracelet, and/or a *I Have Diabetes* ID card in their wallets/purses to help emergency medical personnel treat them properly in emergency situations, from black outs to car accidents. If an Emergency Medical Technician (EMT) or physician found you unconscious and did not know you were a person with diabetes, you might be treated with intravenous glucose—which by itself could put you into diabetic shock or coma.

How Can I Better Control High and Low Blood Sugars?

With the guidance of your diabetes healthcare team, your best bet for prevention of blood sugars that are too high or too low is knowledge and preparation. Know the warning signs of both conditions, and always be prepared to address either one. In addition to always having your blood glucometer nearby for testing, also keep fast-acting sugar near you always, such as in your pocket, your glove compartment, and your briefcase and by your bed, especially if you use insulin. Fast-acting sugars include glucose tablets, glucose gel, or Lifesavers. My personal favorite is the glucose tablets, which are portable and easy to chew up. If you wear dentures and/or take them out at night, a gel or pure fruit juice like orange juice would be a good choice for a low blood sugar emergency.

High and Low Blood Sugar Emergency Information Resources

1. "Hypoglycemia," The American Diabetes Association at *http://www.diabetes.org/living-with-diabetes/treatment-and-care/blood-glucose-control/hypoglycemia-low-blood.html*
2. "Hyperglycemia," The American Diabetes Association, at http://www.diabetes.org/living-with-diabetes/treatment-and-care/blood-glucose-control/hyperglycemia.html

Reviewed by: **Jay Krakovitz, M.D.,** for:

DIABETES SELF-DEFENSE, LLC
6360 Quail Street, Denver, CO 80004
Cell: 303-931-9710; **Web:** www.DiabetesSelfDefense.com

Week Beginning: _____

Weekly Record

MON:	Time	Bld Sgr	Meals	Net Carbs(g)	2 Hrs Bld Sgr	Blood Press	Exercise/Min	Notes/Sickness
Breakfast								
Lunch								
Dinner								
Bedtime								

TUES:	Time	Bld Sgr	Meals	Net Carbs(g)	2 Hrs Bld Sgr	Blood Press	Exercise/Min	Notes/Sickness
Breakfast								
Lunch								
Dinner								
Bedtime								

WED:	Time	Bld Sgr	Meals	Net Carbs(g)	2 Hrs Bld Sgr	Blood Press	Exercise/Min	Notes/Sickness
Breakfast								
Lunch								
Dinner								
Bedtime								

THUR:	Time	Bld Sgr	Meals	Net Carbs(g)	2 Hrs Bld Sgr	Blood Press	Exercise/Min	Notes/Sickness
Breakfast								
Lunch								
Dinner								
Bedtime								

FRI:	Time	Bld Sgr	Meals	Net Carbs(g)	2 Hrs Bld Sgr	Blood Press	Exercise/Min	Notes/Sickness
Breakfast								
Lunch								
Dinner								
Bedtime								

SAT:	Time	Bld Sgr	Meals	Net Carbs(g)	2 Hrs Bld Sgr	Blood Press	Exercise/Min	Notes/Sickness
Breakfast								
Lunch								
Dinner								
Bedtime								

SUN:	Time	Bld Sgr	Meals	Net Carbs(g)	2 Hrs Bld Sgr	Blood Press	Exercise/Min	Notes/Sickness
Breakfast								
Lunch								
Dinner								
Bedtime								

Week 30:
Prescription Medicines for Diabetes

What Does Science Say about Diabetes Prescription Medications?

While a relatively small percentage of people with diabetes (2 percent) are able to control their blood sugar, blood pressure, and cholesterol with diet and exercise alone, the vast majority need prescription medications to help them, and many times multiple prescription medications are needed. Because of this, it is critical for the patient with diabetes to clearly understand any drug interactions and side effects that any given drug may have. Once your doctor prescribes certain medications, you should make sure that every member of your healthcare team has a "master chart" of your medications (see Appendix for your own chart).

The main drugs prescribed for diabetes include: (1) *insulin*; (2) *oral diabetes* medications that: (a) stimulate the pancreas under brand names like Glucotrol®, Prandin®, and Starlix®; (b) suppress the release of sugar by the liver like metformin (Glucophage®); (c) improve the body's sensitivity to insulin and/or lower the amount of sugar released by the liver like Januvia® and Onglyza®; (d) delay the absorption and breakdown of carbohydrates in the intestinal tract like Glyset® and Precose®; (e) offer fixed combinations of the above drugs like Glucovance®, Janumet®, or MetaGlip®; or (3) *injectable diabetes medications* that increase the release of insulin the body produces like Victoza® and Byetta®.

Diabetic patients are also often given prescriptions for other medical problems like ACE inhibitors (Altace®) for blood pressure and cholesterol-lowering drugs like statins (Zocor®, Lipitor®). Unfortunately, all oral diabetes, blood pressure, and cholesterol medications can lose their effectiveness over time, so your doctor may end up changing and/or combining some of your medicines. Different drugs act differently and interact differently with other drugs, foods, and certain dietary supplements. *Make sure you know all the ins and outs of your prescribed medications.* And last, but not least, *never stop taking any prescribed medicine without first telling your doctor.* Stopping certain prescribed medicines like beta blockers, unless you have experienced immediate side effects like nausea and vomiting, can be extremely dangerous and result in coma or death.

How Can I Safely Take My Prescription Medicines for Diabetes/Blood Pressure/High Cholesterol?

Most doctors will keep a careful watch on you when they initially prescribe any new FDA-approved drug for treating your diabetes, blood pressure or high cholesterol; they will take into account all of the medications you are already taking. If you experience any uncomfortable side effects in the first few days, they will ask you to let them know, and then they will discontinue that drug and substitute another that can accomplish the same objective with fewer or no side effects. Like any other part of diabetes management, it is up to you to let your doctor know immediately if you experience side effects like cramps or nausea when you start taking a new diabetes, blood pressure, or cholesterol medication or when your doctor adjusts your dosage.

Diabetes and Prescription Medicine Information Resources

1. Your Primary Care Physician/Diabetes Healthcare Team
2. Aetna Insurance's Consumer Health information at www.intelihealth.com or www.safemedication.com
3. The National Institute of Diabetes and Digestive and Kidney Diseases—*Medicines for People with Diabetes* http://diabetes.niddk.nih.gov/dm/pubs/medicines_ez/

Reviewed by: **Jay Krakovitz, M.D.,** for:

DIABETES SELF-DEFENSE, LLC
6360 Quail Street, Denver, CO 80004
Cell: 303-931-9710; **Web:** www.DiabetesSelfDefense.com

Week Beginning: _____

Weekly Record

MON:	Time	Bld Sgr	Meals	Net Carbs(g)	2 Hrs Bld Sgr	Blood Press	Exercise/Min	Notes/Sickness
Breakfast								
Lunch								
Dinner								
Bedtime								

TUES:	Time	Bld Sgr	Meals	Net Carbs(g)	2 Hrs Bld Sgr	Blood Press	Exercise/Min	Notes/Sickness
Breakfast								
Lunch								
Dinner								
Bedtime								

WED:	Time	Bld Sgr	Meals	Net Carbs(g)	2 Hrs Bld Sgr	Blood Press	Exercise/Min	Notes/Sickness
Breakfast								
Lunch								
Dinner								
Bedtime								

THUR:	Time	Bld Sgr	Meals	Net Carbs(g)	2 Hrs Bld Sgr	Blood Press	Exercise/Min	Notes/Sickness
Breakfast								
Lunch								
Dinner								
Bedtime								

FRI:	Time	Bld Sgr	Meals	Net Carbs(g)	2 Hrs Bld Sgr	Blood Press	Exercise/Min	Notes/Sickness
Breakfast								
Lunch								
Dinner								
Bedtime								

SAT:	Time	Bld Sgr	Meals	Net Carbs(g)	2 Hrs Bld Sgr	Blood Press	Exercise/Min	Notes/Sickness
Breakfast								
Lunch								
Dinner								
Bedtime								

SUN:	Time	Bld Sgr	Meals	Net Carbs(g)	2 Hrs Bld Sgr	Blood Press	Exercise/Min	Notes/Sickness
Breakfast								
Lunch								
Dinner								
Bedtime								

Week 31:
Insulin Therapy and Diabetes

What Does Science Say about Insulin Therapy and Diabetes?

Science says that if your pancreas no longer makes enough of the hormone insulin, as in Type 1 diabetes, then you need to take insulin as a shot. You inject the insulin just under the skin with a small, short needle or have the insulin infused with an insulin pump. People with Type 1 diabetes require daily insulin shots for survival; however, up to 40 percent of people with Type 2 diabetes eventually need insulin shots in addition to their oral medications to keep their blood sugar under control.

Insulin lowers blood sugar by moving sugar from the blood into the cells of your body. Once inside the cells, sugar provides energy. Insulin lowers your blood sugar whether you eat or not. You should eat on time if you take insulin, or you will risk having a dangerous hypoglycemic or low blood sugar reaction. If your doctor prescribes insulin, you should also plan to always *be prepared* for a potential low blood sugar reaction in case you haven't eaten enough; one way is to always have enough fast-acting sugar with you like glucose tablets or LifeSavers.

What Are the Main Types of Insulin?

There are five main types of insulin as listed below. They each work at different speeds. Many people take two types of insulin, usually a fast-acting insulin and a slower acting insulin.

Insulin Type	Action Begins	Peak	Duration
Short-acting	30 minutes–1 hour	2-4 hours	6-8 hours
Rapid acting	10-15 minutes	2 hours	4 hours
Intermediate-acting	1-4 hours	6-12 hours	12-24 hours
Long-acting	4-6 hours	18-28 hours	22-36 hours
Mixtures	Varies, based on mix	Varies, based on mix	Varies

How Can I Manage Insulin Properly?

Most people with insulin-dependent diabetes need at least two insulin shots a day for good blood sugar control. Some people take three or four shots a day to have a more flexible diabetes plan. Today's short needles have such fine gauges that they are virtually painless. You can also check out insulin pumps in the ADA's resource guide. You should take insulin thirty minutes before a meal if you take regular insulin alone or with a longer-acting insulin. If you take a rapid-acting insulin, you should take your shot just before you eat.

Never take a very-rapid or rapid-acting insulin if you're not planning to eat soon. If you begin to feel shaky or sweaty even if you've eaten, test your blood sugar. Some people cannot tell when or *feel* when their blood sugar drops too low, a condition known as hypoglycemia unawareness. If in doubt, test!

Diabetes and Insulin Information Resources

1. The National Institute of Diabetes and Digestive and Kidney Diseases www.niddk.nih.gov
2. Eli Lilly and Company, www.LillyDiabetes.com
3. What You Need To Know About Insulin at http://www.endocrineweb.com/guides/insulin/what-you-need-know-About-insulin

Reviewed by: **Jay Krakovitz, M.D.,** for:

DIABETES SELF-DEFENSE, LLC
6360 Quail Street, Denver, CO 80004
Cell: 303-931-9710; **Web:** www.DiabetesSelfDefense.com

Week Beginning: _____

Weekly Record

MON:	Time	Bld Sgr	Meals	Net Carbs(g)	2 Hrs Bld Sgr	Blood Press	Exercise/Min	Notes/Sickness
Breakfast								
Lunch								
Dinner								
Bedtime								

TUES:	Time	Bld Sgr	Meals	Net Carbs(g)	2 Hrs Bld Sgr	Blood Press	Exercise/Min	Notes/Sickness
Breakfast								
Lunch								
Dinner								
Bedtime								

WED:	Time	Bld Sgr	Meals	Net Carbs(g)	2 Hrs Bld Sgr	Blood Press	Exercise/Min	Notes/Sickness
Breakfast								
Lunch								
Dinner								
Bedtime								

THUR:	Time	Bld Sgr	Meals	Net Carbs(g)	2 Hrs Bld Sgr	Blood Press	Exercise/Min	Notes/Sickness
Breakfast								
Lunch								
Dinner								
Bedtime								

FRI:	Time	Bld Sgr	Meals	Net Carbs(g)	2 Hrs Bld Sgr	Blood Press	Exercise/Min	Notes/Sickness
Breakfast								
Lunch								
Dinner								
Bedtime								

SAT:	Time	Bld Sgr	Meals	Net Carbs(g)	2 Hrs Bld Sgr	Blood Press	Exercise/Min	Notes/Sickness
Breakfast								
Lunch								
Dinner								
Bedtime								

SUN:	Time	Bld Sgr	Meals	Net Carbs(g)	2 Hrs Bld Sgr	Blood Press	Exercise/Min	Notes/Sickness
Breakfast								
Lunch								
Dinner								
Bedtime								

Week 32:
Over-the-Counter (OTC) Medicines and Diabetes

What Does Science Say about Diabetes and OTC Medicines?

Everyday illnesses like coughs, colds, and heartburn affect people with diabetes just like everyone else, but people with diabetes must be very careful when choosing their OTC medicines. The reason? Many OTC medications for everyday illnesses can create major health issues for people with diabetes—such as raising blood sugar and/or blood pressure. Moreover, many of these products can also interact with your prescription diabetes medications, making them much stronger or weaker than intended by your physician.

That's why it's always best to check with your doctor or pharmacist before taking any OTC medications for conditions like coughs, colds, flu, heartburn, etc. The simple fact is that certain OTC medications—while essentially harmless to the non-diabetic general population—can damage kidneys, increase or decrease blood sugar and even cause death.

Why Should I Be Concerned about OTC Medications?

In general, FDA packaging regulations require all manufacturers to label their OTC drug products with any contraindications (side effects) and drug interactions. This simply means that you need to read all OTC drug labels carefully, even if they are in small type. There are many OTC drugs that contain added sugar, alcohol, and/or pseudoephedrine, which can raise blood sugar and blood pressure and should be avoided. Note: non-steroidal anti-inflammatory drugs or NSAIDS like Motrin IB®, Ibuprofen, Advil®, and Aleve® can cause a decrease of blood flow to the kidneys, which can cause a worsening of kidney function in those who have kidney problems or are on dialysis.

How Should I Choose OTC Medicines if I Have Diabetes?

Your best defense against side effects and drug interactions is *knowledge*. You can check out most OTC product safety/side effects/interactions at www.intelihealth.com or www.safemedication.com by directly consulting with your doctor or pharmacist. Just like with prescription drugs, you need to read the label closely before taking anything. Some of the more popular diabetes-friendly (sugar-free, pseudoephedrine-free) medications include:

- *Cough Drops*: N'ice®; Diabetic Tussin®; Ricola®; Fisherman's Friend®
- *Cough Medicine*: Diabetic Tussin® DM; Robitussin® Sugar-Free
- *Allergies*: Diabetic Tussin® AL Allergy Relief
- *Colds*: Cold-Eeze® Sugar-Free Cold Medication; Coricidin HBP
- *Headaches*: Bayer® or generic aspirin; acetaminophen (Tylenol)
- *Sore Throat*: Chloroseptic® Throat Spray
- *Antacids*: Be careful as most are loaded with sodium; Tums® sugar-free is okay
- *Diarrhea*: Generic loperamide is okay

OTC Medications and Diabetes Information Resources

1. "What Ails You? If you have diabetes, some over-the-counter cold and cough medicines can do more harm than good," *Diabetes Forecast*, February, 2003
2. The National Kidney Foundation www.kidney.org
3. www.intelihealth.com or www.safemedication.com

Week Beginning: _____

Weekly Record

MON:	Time	Bld Sgr	Meals	Net Carbs(g)	2 Hrs Bld Sgr	Blood Press	Exercise/Min	Notes/Sickness
Breakfast								
Lunch								
Dinner								
Bedtime								

TUES:	Time	Bld Sgr	Meals	Net Carbs(g)	2 Hrs Bld Sgr	Blood Press	Exercise/Min	Notes/Sickness
Breakfast								
Lunch								
Dinner								
Bedtime								

WED:	Time	Bld Sgr	Meals	Net Carbs(g)	2 Hrs Bld Sgr	Blood Press	Exercise/Min	Notes/Sickness
Breakfast								
Lunch								
Dinner								
Bedtime								

THUR:	Time	Bld Sgr	Meals	Net Carbs(g)	2 Hrs Bld Sgr	Blood Press	Exercise/Min	Notes/Sickness
Breakfast								
Lunch								
Dinner								
Bedtime								

FRI:	Time	Bld Sgr	Meals	Net Carbs(g)	2 Hrs Bld Sgr	Blood Press	Exercise/Min	Notes/Sickness
Breakfast								
Lunch								
Dinner								
Bedtime								

SAT:	Time	Bld Sgr	Meals	Net Carbs(g)	2 Hrs Bld Sgr	Blood Press	Exercise/Min	Notes/Sickness
Breakfast								
Lunch								
Dinner								
Bedtime								

SUN:	Time	Bld Sgr	Meals	Net Carbs(g)	2 Hrs Bld Sgr	Blood Press	Exercise/Min	Notes/Sickness
Breakfast								
Lunch								
Dinner								
Bedtime								

Week 33:
New Aspirin Guidelines for Diabetes Patients

What Does Science Say about Aspirin Therapy and Diabetes?

The following article was published in *Science Daily* on June 2, 2010:

> Experts are now recommending that low-dose aspirin therapy to prevent heart attacks be used somewhat more conservatively—that men younger than fifty and women younger than sixty, who have diabetes but no other major risk factors, probably not use aspirin.
>
> The new recommendations are based on an analysis of nine studies, which found that the risks of some side effects such as stomach bleeding, and to a much less extent bleeding strokes, have to be better balanced against the potential benefits of using aspirin.

Researchers said there is no evidence that higher doses of aspirin beyond the range of 75-162 milligrams per day have any added value in preventing heart attacks. An adequate level of protection is generally achieved with what's considered a "baby aspirin," usually sold in the U.S. as a pill of 81 milligrams, or one-fourth the strength of a typical 325 milligram single aspirin pill.

"Additional studies in patients with diabetes are being conducted to further demonstrate exactly who would best benefit from aspirin therapy," Williams said.

How Should I Use the Latest Aspirin Guidelines If I Have Diabetes?

Discuss aspirin use with your primary care doctor, who will be able to take into account your unique condition and current medication plan. You may also want to discuss aspirin use with your cardiologist, if you have one, for heart health. Whether or not to take aspirin—and in what specific doses—is something that should come from your doctor, not from the latest findings posted on the internet.

Aspirin and Diabetes Information Resources

1. "New Aspirin Guidelines For Diabetes Patients," Hendrick, Bill, June 2, 2010, http://diabetes.webmd.com/news/20100602/new-aspirin-guidelines-for-diabetes-patients?print=true
2. "Aspirin Recommendations Changed for Many Younger Diabetic Patients," *June 2, 2010*, http://www.sciencedaily.com/releases/2010/06/100601162251.htm

Reviewed by: **Jay Krakovitz, M.D.,** for:

DIABETES SELF-DEFENSE, LLC
6360 Quail Street, Denver, CO 80004
Cell: 303-931-9710; **Web:** www.DiabetesSelfDefense.com

Week Beginning: _____

Weekly Record

MON:	Time	Bld Sgr	Meals	Net Carbs(g)	2 Hrs Bld Sgr	Blood Press	Exercise/Min	Notes/Sickness
Breakfast								
Lunch								
Dinner								
Bedtime								

TUES:	Time	Bld Sgr	Meals	Net Carbs(g)	2 Hrs Bld Sgr	Blood Press	Exercise/Min	Notes/Sickness
Breakfast								
Lunch								
Dinner								
Bedtime								

WED:	Time	Bld Sgr	Meals	Net Carbs(g)	2 Hrs Bld Sgr	Blood Press	Exercise/Min	Notes/Sickness
Breakfast								
Lunch								
Dinner								
Bedtime								

THUR:	Time	Bld Sgr	Meals	Net Carbs(g)	2 Hrs Bld Sgr	Blood Press	Exercise/Min	Notes/Sickness
Breakfast								
Lunch								
Dinner								
Bedtime								

FRI:	Time	Bld Sgr	Meals	Net Carbs(g)	2 Hrs Bld Sgr	Blood Press	Exercise/Min	Notes/Sickness
Breakfast								
Lunch								
Dinner								
Bedtime								

SAT:	Time	Bld Sgr	Meals	Net Carbs(g)	2 Hrs Bld Sgr	Blood Press	Exercise/Min	Notes/Sickness
Breakfast								
Lunch								
Dinner								
Bedtime								

SUN:	Time	Bld Sgr	Meals	Net Carbs(g)	2 Hrs Bld Sgr	Blood Press	Exercise/Min	Notes/Sickness
Breakfast								
Lunch								
Dinner								
Bedtime								

Week 34:
Diabetes and Sick Days

What Does Science Say about Sick Days for People with Diabetes?

Science tells us that people with diabetes, because of their compromised immune systems, have very different needs than non-diabetics on sick days. It's very important to take care of yourself when you're sick as many types of illness stress can drive up your blood sugar levels, including even the common cold. *Never take any prescription or OTC medicine without your doctor's approval, and remember to carefully read the instructions on all medications as most medicines are not intended for people with diabetes and may cause serious side effects.* When in doubt about the best medicine to take for your illness, such as a cough or cold, check with your doctor or pharmacist. If the medicine is not recommended for people with diabetes, it will say so on the label.

More and more, though, some medicines are being made specifically for people with diabetes. When you're sick, here are some good general guidelines: (1) Check your blood sugar every four hours and write down the results; (2) Keep taking your insulin and your diabetes pills. Even if you can't keep food down, you still need your diabetes medicine. Ask your doctor or diabetes educator whether to change the amount of insulin or pills you take; (3) Drink at least a cup (eight ounces) of water or other calorie-free, caffeine-free liquid every hour while you're awake; (4) If you can't eat your usual food, try drinking juice or eating crackers, popsicles, or soup; (5) If you can't eat at all, drink clear liquids such as ginger ale. Eat or drink something with sugar in it if you have trouble keeping food down; (6) Test your urine for ketones if your blood sugar is over 240 mg/dL or if you can't keep food or liquids down.

However, call your health care provider *right away* if: (1) your blood sugar has been over 240 mg/dL for longer than a day; (2) you have moderate to large amounts of ketones in your urine; (3) you feel sleepier than usual; (4) you have trouble breathing; (5) you can't think clearly; (6) you throw up more than once; (7) you've had diarrhea for more than six hours.

How Should I Manage Diabetes Sick Days?

For everyday sicknesses like coughs, colds, upset stomach, and headaches, make sure you have diabetes-friendly OTC (over-the-counter) medications. There are many OTC medicines that should not be taken by people with diabetes. Always read the package labels carefully as they will have warnings, if required, for people with diabetes; in addition to looking at the list of *active ingredients* that can affect your blood sugar or blood pressure—for example, *pseudoephedrine*, *phenylpropanolamine*, and *phenylephrine* are decongestants that can raise blood pressure—you need to look at *inactive ingredients* like added sugar or alcohol that can raise or lower your blood sugar.

Pain medications like aspirin and acetaminophen (Tylenol) are usually okay in small doses. Ibuprofen (Motrin IB or generic ibuprofen), however, is not, as it can cause renal failure in anyone with kidney problems. People with diabetes should not be taking ibuprofen without discussing it first with their doctor.

Diabetes and Sick Days Information Resources

1. BD Diabetes.com, "Sick Days and Diabetes" at http://www.bd.com/us/diabetes/page.aspx?cat=7001&id=7148 and http://www.bd.com/us/diabetes/page.aspx?cat=7001&id=7347
2. The American Diabetes Association, "Sick Days," at http://www.diabetes.org/living-with-diabetes/parents-and-kids/everyday-life/sick-days.html

Part 6:
"T" = Targeted Nutritional Support

"T" Section Summary

While it is certainly true that the dietary supplements industry has exploded in the past few decades in terms of sales, it is equally true that the amount of clinical support for the majority of supplements remains quite small. However, there are a few dietary supplements that are backed by science, and several of these can be a helpful addition to your primary diabetes management program, which has diet, exercise, and medications as its core. Perhaps the most well-known of these helpful supplements are multivitamin/multimineral supplements and the Omega-3 supplements like high-quality fish oil. Finally, one of the best researched, though perhaps least known, of scientifically-supported dietary supplements are those from Rob Keller, MD, one of America's top medical researchers and creator of several powerful products that support the body's production and recycling of glutathione, the body's master antioxidant and "maestro of the immune system" according to another well-known physician, Mark Hyman, MD, author of *The Blood Sugar Solution*. You can find out more about Dr. Keller's supplements at our website, www.DiabetesSelfDefense.com, on the Products page.

Reviewed by: **Jay Krakovitz, M.D.,** for:

DIABETES SELF-DEFENSE, LLC
6360 Quail Street, Denver, CO 80004
Cell: 303-931-9710; **Web:** www.DiabetesSelfDefense.com

Week Beginning: _____

Weekly Record

MON:	Time	Bld Sgr	Meals	Net Carbs(g)	2 Hrs Bld Sgr	Blood Press	Exercise/Min	Notes/Sickness
Breakfast								
Lunch								
Dinner								
Bedtime								

TUES:	Time	Bld Sgr	Meals	Net Carbs(g)	2 Hrs Bld Sgr	Blood Press	Exercise/Min	Notes/Sickness
Breakfast								
Lunch								
Dinner								
Bedtime								

WED:	Time	Bld Sgr	Meals	Net Carbs(g)	2 Hrs Bld Sgr	Blood Press	Exercise/Min	Notes/Sickness
Breakfast								
Lunch								
Dinner								
Bedtime								

THUR:	Time	Bld Sgr	Meals	Net Carbs(g)	2 Hrs Bld Sgr	Blood Press	Exercise/Min	Notes/Sickness
Breakfast								
Lunch								
Dinner								
Bedtime								

FRI:	Time	Bld Sgr	Meals	Net Carbs(g)	2 Hrs Bld Sgr	Blood Press	Exercise/Min	Notes/Sickness
Breakfast								
Lunch								
Dinner								
Bedtime								

SAT:	Time	Bld Sgr	Meals	Net Carbs(g)	2 Hrs Bld Sgr	Blood Press	Exercise/Min	Notes/Sickness
Breakfast								
Lunch								
Dinner								
Bedtime								

SUN:	Time	Bld Sgr	Meals	Net Carbs(g)	2 Hrs Bld Sgr	Blood Press	Exercise/Min	Notes/Sickness
Breakfast								
Lunch								
Dinner								
Bedtime								

Week 35:
Alternative Medicine and Diabetes

What Does Science Say about Alternative Medicine and Diabetes?

Dr. Michael J. Quon, Chief of the Diabetes Unit of the National Center for Complementary and Alternative Medicine (NCCAM), which has been created by the National Institutes of Health, defined complementary and alternative medicine (CAM) as a "medical and health care practice outside the realm of conventional medicine, which is yet to be validated using scientific methods," keeping in mind that it should *complement* conventional practices and/or be an *alternative* to those approaches.

The scope of CAM is very broad, and includes manipulative techniques (massage, chiropractic), mind-body medicine (yoga), energy therapies (magnetic bands), and alternative systems (homeopathy), as well as natural, herbal, and diet-based medicine. Despite disappointing results in initial studies, research into complementary and alternative medicine continues in the context of diabetes and metabolic diseases. NCCAM has initiated specific studies into alternative treatments for diabetes, the metabolic syndrome, and obesity.

Why Should I Consider Alternative Medicine for Diabetes?

While alternative medicine therapies have been used widely around the world for thousands of years for various conditions, diabetes nonetheless represents a great challenge. Scientific support for alternative medicine in fighting diabetes has been limited, but the most promising area is that of natural dietary supplements as a complement to mainstream medicine. However, even *natural* supplements can interact with diabetes medications and have side effects, so always notify you doctor if you begin taking dietary supplements.

According to a study noted below from *Diabetes Care* in 2003, there is still insufficient evidence to draw any final conclusions about the safety and effectiveness of herbs and dietary supplements for blood sugar control, though several have shown positive initial results, including *Gymnema sylvestre* and *American ginseng*. Other dietary supplements have been tested for helping with weight control, high blood pressure, and high cholesterol with very limited levels of success. Even old standbys like garlic supplements for cholesterol have very little scientific support.

How Should I Use Alternative Medicine in My Diabetes Management Plan?

The best starting point with alternative medicine is knowledge. The Harvard Medical School and the Natural Standard, an association of alternative and conventional physicians, have published rigorous reviews of the science and safety of alternative medicine and dietary supplements at www.intelihealth.com, a service of Aetna insurance. By reviewing the information on this site carefully, you can better assess the safety and effectiveness of herbs, dietary supplements, and alternative medicine treatments. In his book, *Reversing Diabetes*, Julian Whitaker, MD, offers support for a series of potential dietary supplements that may be of value in fighting diabetes as part of an overall diabetes management plan. In his 2012 book, *The Blood Sugar Solution*, Mark Hyman, MD, also has a list of nutritional supplements that he suggests to his patients, including glutathione, which Dr. Hyman refers to as "the mother of all antioxidants" and "the most important molecule you need to stay healthy and prevent disease — yet you've probably never heard of it."

Alternative Medicine for Diabetes Information Resources

1. Diabetes and CAM: A Focus On Dietary Supplements, National Center for Complementary and Alternative Medicine at http://www.diabetes.org/living-with-diabetes/treatment-and-care/blood-glucose-control/hypoglycemia-low-blood.html
2. Aetna Insurance's Consumer Health Information website, www.intelihealth.com
3. Hyman, Mark, MD, http://www.huffingtonpost.com/dr-mark-hyman/glutathione-the-mother-of_b_530494.html

Reviewed by: **Jay Krakovitz, M.D.,** for:

DIABETES SELF-DEFENSE, LLC
6360 Quail Street, Denver, CO 80004
Cell: 303-931-9710; **Web:** www.DiabetesSelfDefense.com

Week Beginning: _____

Weekly Record

MON:	Time	Bld Sgr	Meals	Net Carbs(g)	2 Hrs Bld Sgr	Blood Press	Exercise/Min	Notes/Sickness
Breakfast								
Lunch								
Dinner								
Bedtime								

TUES:	Time	Bld Sgr	Meals	Net Carbs(g)	2 Hrs Bld Sgr	Blood Press	Exercise/Min	Notes/Sickness
Breakfast								
Lunch								
Dinner								
Bedtime								

WED:	Time	Bld Sgr	Meals	Net Carbs(g)	2 Hrs Bld Sgr	Blood Press	Exercise/Min	Notes/Sickness
Breakfast								
Lunch								
Dinner								
Bedtime								

THUR:	Time	Bld Sgr	Meals	Net Carbs(g)	2 Hrs Bld Sgr	Blood Press	Exercise/Min	Notes/Sickness
Breakfast								
Lunch								
Dinner								
Bedtime								

FRI:	Time	Bld Sgr	Meals	Net Carbs(g)	2 Hrs Bld Sgr	Blood Press	Exercise/Min	Notes/Sickness
Breakfast								
Lunch								
Dinner								
Bedtime								

SAT:	Time	Bld Sgr	Meals	Net Carbs(g)	2 Hrs Bld Sgr	Blood Press	Exercise/Min	Notes/Sickness
Breakfast								
Lunch								
Dinner								
Bedtime								

SUN:	Time	Bld Sgr	Meals	Net Carbs(g)	2 Hrs Bld Sgr	Blood Press	Exercise/Min	Notes/Sickness
Breakfast								
Lunch								
Dinner								
Bedtime								

Week 36:
Dietary Supplements and Diabetes

What Does Science Say about Dietary Supplements for Diabetes?

The National Center for Complementary and Alternative Medicine (NCCAM), a division of the National Institutes of Health (NIH), has published the following points in its national fact sheet:

- In general, there is not enough scientific evidence to prove that dietary supplements have substantial benefits for Type 2 diabetes or its complications.
- It is very important not to replace conventional medical therapy for diabetes with an unproven complementary/alternative medicine.
- Tell your healthcare provider about any complementary and alternative practices you use. Give them a full picture of what you do to manage your health. This will help ensure coordinated and safe care.
- Some of the dietary supplements currently under scientific review for people with diabetes include alpha lipoic acid, chromium, omega-3 fatty acids, and polyphenols.

That said, our review of the dietary supplement world for people with diabetes or pre-diabetes has revealed one line of supplements that has been scientifically researched and developed by a physician, Rob Keller, MD; more information on Dr. Keller's glutathione-supporting supplements can be found on our website, www. DiabetesSelfDefense.com on the Products page. Dr. Keller's work has been nationally recognized as well as his outstanding contributions to science; Dr. Keller was voted as one of the "top 2000 outstanding scientists" of the 21st century.

Why Should I Be Concerned with Dietary Supplements?

Many nutritional or dietary supplements can interact with prescribed diabetes medications, potentially increasing or decreasing the power of that medication. Therefore, while potentially helpful, they need to be added with great care. Dietary supplements are not regulated for safety and effectiveness by the FDA as are prescription and OTC drugs.

"The Institute of Medicine, a private advisory body to the U.S. government, is calling for tougher regulation of dietary supplements, including quality-control rules and better proof that they work," the Associated Press recently reported. In a report issued January 12, 2005, the institute urged Congress to require supplement makers to prove their products are safe and effective, just as manufacturers of conventional drugs must do now.

How Should I Select Dietary Supplements for My Diabetes Management?

The best starting point with dietary supplements is knowledge. The Harvard Medical School and the Natural Standard, an association of alternative and conventional physicians, have published rigorous reviews of the science and safety of alternative medicine and dietary supplements at www.intelihealth.com, a service of Aetna insurance. By reviewing the information on these sites carefully, you can better assess the safety and effectiveness of herbs, dietary supplements, and alternative medicine treatments. Some of the latest dietary supplements shown to be scientifically effective for people with diabetes include *Omega-3 fish oil* (www.cardiotabs.com), *CoQ10* (especially if you are taking a statin like Lipitor®), and *alpha lipoic acid*. Be sure to discuss the use of dietary supplements with your doctor *before* you add them to your personal diabetes program.

Diabetes and Dietary Supplements Information Resources

1. Yeh, Eisenberg, et al, "Systematic Review of Herbs and Dietary Supplements for Glycemic Control in Diabetes," *Diabetes Care* 26: 1277-1294, 2003.
2. Aetna Insurance's Consumer Health Information website, www.intelihealth.com; *Complementary and Alternative Medicine*
3. The National Center for Complementary and Alternative Medicine, "*C a.m. and Diabetes: A Focus on Dietary Supplements*," at http://nccam.nih.gov/health/diabetes/

Reviewed by: **Jay Krakovitz, M.D.,** for:

DIABETES SELF-DEFENSE, LLC
6360 Quail Street, Denver, CO 80004
Cell: 303-931-9710; **Web:** www.DiabetesSelfDefense.com

Week Beginning: _____

Weekly Record

MON:	Time	Bld Sgr	Meals	Net Carbs(g)	2 Hrs Bld Sgr	Blood Press	Exercise/Min	Notes/Sickness
Breakfast								
Lunch								
Dinner								
Bedtime								

TUES:	Time	Bld Sgr	Meals	Net Carbs(g)	2 Hrs Bld Sgr	Blood Press	Exercise/Min	Notes/Sickness
Breakfast								
Lunch								
Dinner								
Bedtime								

WED:	Time	Bld Sgr	Meals	Net Carbs(g)	2 Hrs Bld Sgr	Blood Press	Exercise/Min	Notes/Sickness
Breakfast								
Lunch								
Dinner								
Bedtime								

THUR:	Time	Bld Sgr	Meals	Net Carbs(g)	2 Hrs Bld Sgr	Blood Press	Exercise/Min	Notes/Sickness
Breakfast								
Lunch								
Dinner								
Bedtime								

FRI:	Time	Bld Sgr	Meals	Net Carbs(g)	2 Hrs Bld Sgr	Blood Press	Exercise/Min	Notes/Sickness
Breakfast								
Lunch								
Dinner								
Bedtime								

SAT:	Time	Bld Sgr	Meals	Net Carbs(g)	2 Hrs Bld Sgr	Blood Press	Exercise/Min	Notes/Sickness
Breakfast								
Lunch								
Dinner								
Bedtime								

SUN:	Time	Bld Sgr	Meals	Net Carbs(g)	2 Hrs Bld Sgr	Blood Press	Exercise/Min	Notes/Sickness
Breakfast								
Lunch								
Dinner								
Bedtime								

Week 37:
"Special Foods" for Diabetes

What Does Science Say about "Special Foods" for Diabetes?

Any foods that can help an individual better control their weight, blood sugar, blood pressure, and cholesterol would be beneficial, regardless of the presence of diabetes or not. For people with diabetes, it is critical to their well-being to control these variables. Scientific research has recently shown that there are certain foods, that, when consumed in moderation within a diabetes meal plan, can help people with diabetes lose weight and gain better control of their blood sugar, blood pressure, and cholesterol.

Science has also shown us that the key to getting control and keeping control is not simply a matter of eating the right foods in the right portion sizes, but to do that *and* to get an adequate amount of moderate exercise or activity each day—whether gardening, walking, swimming, or jogging, etc. So while a healthy diet is critical for effective diabetes management, it is not sufficient in and of itself to help the person with diabetes gain and maintain diabetes control—you also need regular activity to improve your metabolism.

Why Should I Consider Using "Special Foods" for Diabetes?

While there is nothing magic about any certain food for people with diabetes, nor is there anything magic or uniquely beneficial from sugar-free, diabetic foods, there are a few foods that are scientifically supported in their ability to help with diabetes control: Glucerna® shakes and bars, phytosterol/stanol margarines like Take Control® and Smart Balance®; glucomannan foods, and Salba® Seeds (www.salba.com). Glucomannan, which is from the root of a plant in Asia and is pure soluble fiber, is readily available as pasta and/or powder forms. Both Take Control® and Benecol® margarine spreads have been scientifically shown to help promote healthy cholesterol levels when eaten as part of a low-fat, low-cholesterol diet; the FDA authorized their cholesterol-lowering claims based on evidence that the plant sterol and stanol esters in these products may help lower LDL—bad—cholesterol, without affecting HDL—good—cholesterol, reducing the risk of coronary heart disease in some individuals. Salba® Seeds are a new entry into the market, but they provide a very powerful nutritional package. In his latest book, *The Sugar Blockers Diet*, Rob Thompson, MD, reveals several nutritional strategies for helping improve blood sugar control, strategies that incorporate the use of several everyday foods.

How Should I Incorporate These Special Foods into My Diabetes Meal Plan?

While many of the above foods are readily available at your local supermarket, there are a few companies that offer very special versions of glucomannan (www.konjacfoods.com) or Miracle Noodle at www.miraclenoodle.com.

You can also find out more about Salba® Seeds and the science behind them at www.salba.com. Never forget, though, that *special foods* should always be an addition to a healthy meal plan, not a replacement. For people with diabetes looking to develop a sound, well-balanced meal plan, I strongly recommend that you read *The Low-Starch Diabetes Solution* and/or *The Sugar Blockers Diet* by Rob Thompson, MD, to see which fits best into your lifestyle.

Special Foods for Diabetes Information Resources

1. "Salba The Seed of Wellness: An Ancient Grain That is Chasing Diabetes," *at http://www.salba.com/system/articles/1/original/2009_03_Diabetes_Communicator.pdf?1244738792*
2. Vuksan, et al, "Konjac-mannan (glucomannan) improves glycemia and other associated risk factors for coronary heart disease in type 2 diabetes. A randomized controlled metabolic trial," *Diabetes Care*, 1999 Jun; 22(6):913-9.
3. Thompson, Rob, MD, *The Sugar Blockers Diet*, http://www.amazon.com/The-Sugar-Blockers-Diet-Diabetes/dp/1609618432

Part 7:
"S" = Study Diabetes!

"S" Section Overview

Like any other subject you want to understand better, the more you study, the more you learn. Diabetes is no different in that respect, but unlike other major diseases, control of diabetes rests very heavily on the shoulders of the patient. This is why we firmly believe that in the War Against Diabetes, *the ultimate weapon is knowledge*. New information arrives every day in the world of diabetes, and what is popular one day may be out of favor the next. The way diabetes is managed today is drastically different than it was only ten to fifteen years ago as a result of new discoveries and new information. And while new information is important, it is also critical that people with diabetes are well-versed in the basics of diabetes management. Just as when you were in school and learned from many different teachers/professors, so it is in the world of diabetes education—you must listen to the different experts and apply that knowledge to your own unique situation.

Reviewed by: **Jay Krakovitz, M.D.,** for:

DIABETES SELF-DEFENSE, LLC
6360 Quail Street, Denver, CO 80004
Cell: 303-931-9710; **Web:** www.DiabetesSelfDefense.com

Week Beginning: _____

Weekly Record

MON:	Time	Bld Sgr	Meals	Net Carbs(g)	2 Hrs Bld Sgr	Blood Press	Exercise/Min	Notes/Sickness
Breakfast								
Lunch								
Dinner								
Bedtime								

TUES:	Time	Bld Sgr	Meals	Net Carbs(g)	2 Hrs Bld Sgr	Blood Press	Exercise/Min	Notes/Sickness
Breakfast								
Lunch								
Dinner								
Bedtime								

WED:	Time	Bld Sgr	Meals	Net Carbs(g)	2 Hrs Bld Sgr	Blood Press	Exercise/Min	Notes/Sickness
Breakfast								
Lunch								
Dinner								
Bedtime								

THUR:	Time	Bld Sgr	Meals	Net Carbs(g)	2 Hrs Bld Sgr	Blood Press	Exercise/Min	Notes/Sickness
Breakfast								
Lunch								
Dinner								
Bedtime								

FRI:	Time	Bld Sgr	Meals	Net Carbs(g)	2 Hrs Bld Sgr	Blood Press	Exercise/Min	Notes/Sickness
Breakfast								
Lunch								
Dinner								
Bedtime								

SAT:	Time	Bld Sgr	Meals	Net Carbs(g)	2 Hrs Bld Sgr	Blood Press	Exercise/Min	Notes/Sickness
Breakfast								
Lunch								
Dinner								
Bedtime								

SUN:	Time	Bld Sgr	Meals	Net Carbs(g)	2 Hrs Bld Sgr	Blood Press	Exercise/Min	Notes/Sickness
Breakfast								
Lunch								
Dinner								
Bedtime								

Week 38:
Education and Training for Diabetes

What Does Science Say about Diabetes Education and Training?

National statistics have shown that people with diabetes today have an extremely hard time keeping their "ABCs of diabetes" under control: their *A1C* blood sugar (7 percent or less); their *B*lood Pressure (130/80 or less); and their *C*holesterol (LDL 100 mg/dL or less); in fact, only 7 percent of people with diabetes are able to achieve the recommended health goals for all three. When people with diabetes are trained in diabetes management, generally with the help of a certified diabetes educator (CDE), they do a better job of managing their diabetes and experience fewer complications than those who do not undergo the training.

Diabetes education and training is not only critical when you are initially diagnosed, but it's equally important to stay current with the latest research and diabetes management methods, which can change dramatically in a matter of only a few years. What you and/or your doctor may have learned about diabetes management when you were initially diagnosed—perhaps five, ten, or fifteen years ago—has changed significantly in recent years with the advent of medical technology/research and nutritional science.

Just as your doctor, nutritionist, and diabetes educators are required to stay current in order to maintain their licenses, so should you stay as current as you can on the latest developments in diabetes management. And while the Internet has provided a huge leap in information availability about diabetes, care and caution are needed when using the information found—always check to be sure that the information is scientifically sound and from a highly credible organization.

Why Should I Be Concerned about Diabetes Education and Training?

People with diabetes are at higher than normal risk than the general population for serious diseases related to blood vessel complications, including heart disease, kidney failure, blindness, and nerve disorders. Research shows that diabetes patients that receive education on a regular basis gain better control of their diabetes than those that do not receive such training. One of the most recent and dramatic demonstrations of this fact took place in Arkansas in 2004 with the *Arkansas Diabetes Control Program*, a program that produced dramatic improvements in diabetic Medicaid patients control of their blood sugar and blood pressure thanks to an aggressive patient education program. In summary, diabetes education works!

How Can I Get the Best Diabetes Education and Training?

To find a certified diabetes educator in your area, visit the American Association of Diabetes Educators at their website at www.diabeteseducator.org and type in your zip code; a list of certified diabetes educators in your area will appear. You can also check with your local hospital to see what type, if any, of diabetes support groups they provide. Many hospitals have diabetes support groups that meet on a monthly basis.

Education and Training for Diabetes Information Resources

1. The American Association of Diabetes Educators www.diabeteseducator.org
2. Arkansas Diabetes Control Program at http://www.healthy.arkansas.gov/programsServices/chronic Disease/diabetesPreventionControl/Pages/default.aspx.
3. Johns Hopkins University, "New Diabetes Education Yields Better Control," at http://gazette.jhu.edu/2011/04/18/new-diabetes-education-yields-improved-blood-sugar-control/

Reviewed by: **Jay Krakovitz, M.D.,** for:

DIABETES SELF-DEFENSE, LLC
6360 Quail Street, Denver, CO 80004
Cell: 303-931-9710; **Web:** www.DiabetesSelfDefense.com

Week Beginning: _____

Weekly Record

MON:	Time	Bld Sgr	Meals	Net Carbs(g)	2 Hrs Bld Sgr	Blood Press	Exercise/Min	Notes/Sickness
Breakfast								
Lunch								
Dinner								
Bedtime								

TUES:	Time	Bld Sgr	Meals	Net Carbs(g)	2 Hrs Bld Sgr	Blood Press	Exercise/Min	Notes/Sickness
Breakfast								
Lunch								
Dinner								
Bedtime								

WED:	Time	Bld Sgr	Meals	Net Carbs(g)	2 Hrs Bld Sgr	Blood Press	Exercise/Min	Notes/Sickness
Breakfast								
Lunch								
Dinner								
Bedtime								

THUR:	Time	Bld Sgr	Meals	Net Carbs(g)	2 Hrs Bld Sgr	Blood Press	Exercise/Min	Notes/Sickness
Breakfast								
Lunch								
Dinner								
Bedtime								

FRI:	Time	Bld Sgr	Meals	Net Carbs(g)	2 Hrs Bld Sgr	Blood Press	Exercise/Min	Notes/Sickness
Breakfast								
Lunch								
Dinner								
Bedtime								

SAT:	Time	Bld Sgr	Meals	Net Carbs(g)	2 Hrs Bld Sgr	Blood Press	Exercise/Min	Notes/Sickness
Breakfast								
Lunch								
Dinner								
Bedtime								

SUN:	Time	Bld Sgr	Meals	Net Carbs(g)	2 Hrs Bld Sgr	Blood Press	Exercise/Min	Notes/Sickness
Breakfast								
Lunch								
Dinner								
Bedtime								

Week 39:
Heart Disease and Diabetes

What Does Science Say about Diabetes and Heart Disease?

The largest health threat faced by people with diabetes is the threat of artery disease or atherosclerosis, also known as hardening of the arteries. Artery damage can lead to heart attack, stroke, and sometimes a need for amputations caused by inadequate circulation in the legs. Diabetics are two to four times more likely than non-diabetics to have a heart attack or a stroke. Many diabetics have a family member who has had a heart attack or stroke at a young age, placing them in a known risk group for heart disease before diabetes is even diagnosed.

But family history is only one of several heart risks that are common among diabetics. Why are diabetics so prone to artery disease? Diabetes or too much sugar in the blood over a long period of time contributes to artery disease directly, yet it rarely works alone. People with diabetes are more likely than others to have or to develop additional heart disease risk factors (such as high blood pressure, obesity, smoking, inactive lifestyle, a high fat diet, and high cholesterol). When it comes to heart-disease risks, people with diabetes commonly receive an unfortunate *package deal*, so that instead of one heart-disease risk factor, they have multiple risk factors.

Why Should I Be Concerned about Heart Disease?

Cardiovascular disease (CVD) is the leading cause of death among people with diabetes as it accounts for nearly two out of three deaths. When arteries become clogged and narrowed, you may have one or more heart problems: Chest pain, also called *angina*; *heart attack*; or *cardiomyopathy*. When you have angina, you feel pain in your chest, arms, shoulders, or back. You may feel the pain more when your heart works faster, such as when you exercise. The pain may go away when you rest. You also may feel very weak and sweaty. If you do not get it treated, chest pain may happen more often.

If diabetes has damaged the heart nerves, you may not feel the chest pain. A *heart attack* happens when a blood vessel in or near the heart becomes blocked. Not enough blood can get to that part of the heart muscle. That area of the heart muscle stops working, so the heart is weaker. During a heart attack, you may have chest pain along with nausea, indigestion, extreme weakness, and sweating. *Cardiomyopathy* happens when narrowed blood vessels let less blood flow through the heart. This damage makes the heart muscle weak.

How Can I Prevent Heart Disease and Blood Vessel Problems?

To help prevent heart disease and blood vessel problems, the National Institute for Diabetes, Digestive and Kidney Disorders (NIDDK) recommends the following: keep your blood sugar and blood pressure as close to normal as you can; quit smoking; get About thirty minutes of physical activity or exercise each day; keep blood cholesterol and other blood fats as close to normal as you can; take your diabetes medicines at the same times each day; take your heart pills and blood pressure pills as your doctor tells you; ask your doctor if you should take an aspirin each day to help protect your heart; and follow the healthy eating plan you work out with your doctor or dietitian that is low in saturated fat, sugar, and sodium while high in fiber (with plenty of fruits, vegetables, and whole grains).

Diabetes and Heart Disease Information Resources

1. The National Institute of Diabetes and Digestive and Kidney Diseases http://diabetes.niddk.nih.gov/dm/pubs/complications_heart/
2. The American Diabetes Association, Heart Disease, at http://www.diabetes.org/living-with-diabetes/complications/heart-disease/

Reviewed by: **Jay Krakovitz, M.D.,** for:

DIABETES SELF-DEFENSE, LLC
6360 Quail Street, Denver, CO 80004
Cell: 303-931-9710; **Web:** www.DiabetesSelfDefense.com

Week Beginning: _____

Weekly Record

MON:	Time	Bld Sgr	Meals	Net Carbs(g)	2 Hrs Bld Sgr	Blood Press	Exercise/Min	Notes/Sickness
Breakfast								
Lunch								
Dinner								
Bedtime								

TUES:	Time	Bld Sgr	Meals	Net Carbs(g)	2 Hrs Bld Sgr	Blood Press	Exercise/Min	Notes/Sickness
Breakfast								
Lunch								
Dinner								
Bedtime								

WED:	Time	Bld Sgr	Meals	Net Carbs(g)	2 Hrs Bld Sgr	Blood Press	Exercise/Min	Notes/Sickness
Breakfast								
Lunch								
Dinner								
Bedtime								

THUR:	Time	Bld Sgr	Meals	Net Carbs(g)	2 Hrs Bld Sgr	Blood Press	Exercise/Min	Notes/Sickness
Breakfast								
Lunch								
Dinner								
Bedtime								

FRI:	Time	Bld Sgr	Meals	Net Carbs(g)	2 Hrs Bld Sgr	Blood Press	Exercise/Min	Notes/Sickness
Breakfast								
Lunch								
Dinner								
Bedtime								

SAT:	Time	Bld Sgr	Meals	Net Carbs(g)	2 Hrs Bld Sgr	Blood Press	Exercise/Min	Notes/Sickness
Breakfast								
Lunch								
Dinner								
Bedtime								

SUN:	Time	Bld Sgr	Meals	Net Carbs(g)	2 Hrs Bld Sgr	Blood Press	Exercise/Min	Notes/Sickness
Breakfast								
Lunch								
Dinner								
Bedtime								

Week 40:
Stroke and Diabetes

What Does Science Say about Stroke and Diabetes?

Diabetes significantly increases your risk of having a stroke. A stroke is known medically as an event that occurs when the brain is not getting enough oxygen via the blood, causing part of it to shut down. When it shuts down, certain body functions stop as well, often causing a partial or complete paralysis. People with diabetes are two to four times as likely as non-diabetics to have a stroke as well as to have more debilitating strokes, yet most people with diabetes do not know it. A survey commissioned in 2002 by the American Diabetes Association (ADA) and the American College of Cardiology (ACC) revealed a serious disconnect among people with diabetes about their risk of cardiovascular disease.

The results of the survey revealed that nearly *70 percent* of the more than 2,000 patients surveyed did not even consider cardiovascular disease to be a serious risk associated with their diabetes. A stroke happens when part of your brain is not getting enough blood and stops working. Depending on the part of the brain that is damaged, a stroke can cause: sudden weakness or numbness of your face, arm, or leg on one side of your body; sudden confusion, trouble talking, or trouble understanding; sudden dizziness, loss of balance, or trouble walking; sudden trouble seeing in one or both eyes or sudden double vision; or sudden severe headache. Sometimes, one or more of these warning signs may happen and then disappear. You might be having a "mini-stroke," also called a TIA (transient ischemic attack). If you have any of these warning signs, tell your doctor right away or call 911.

Why Should I Be Concerned about Stroke?

Stroke or cerebral accidents are one of the leading causes of death in America, following close behind heart disease and cancer. Strokes can partially or completely disable an individual as well as cause death. People with diabetes are at higher risk than the general population due to the fact that they have higher risk of heart or blood vessel problems and high blood pressure. However, a study at the Boston University School of Public Health and Medicine, as published at the January, 2003, ADA web site, showed that people with diabetes not only usually have higher blood pressure than non-diabetics, but that *they also receive less aggressive medical treatment than non-diabetics.*

As a result, the researchers from the study concluded:

> There is an urgent need to improve hypertension care and blood pressure control in patients with diabetes. Additional information is required to understand why clinicians are not more aggressive in managing blood pressure when patients also have diabetes.

How Can I Prevent a Stroke?

As with other forms of diabetes management, keeping your blood sugar (80-120 mg/dL) and blood pressure (130/80 or less) in check along with losing excess weight will help prevent damage to your eyes, kidneys, heart, and blood vessels. If possible, you need to quit or minimize smoking and drink alcohol only in moderation (no more than two drinks per day). Additionally, it is important to monitor your blood fats like cholesterol (LDL less than 100 mg/dL) and triglycerides (less than 150 mg/dL) as well. In short, you need to pay close attention to the *ABCs of diabetes* and have daily exercise or activity for twenty minutes or more to help keep excess weight from coming back.

Diabetes and Stroke Information Resources

1. The American Stroke Association or at http://www.heart.org/HEARTORG/Conditions/Diabetes/Diabetes_UCM_001091_SubHomePage.jsp

Reviewed by: **Jay Krakovitz, M.D.,** for:

DIABETES SELF-DEFENSE, LLC
6360 Quail Street, Denver, CO 80004
Cell: 303-931-9710; **Web:** www.DiabetesSelfDefense.com

Week Beginning: _____

Weekly Record

MON:	Time	Bld Sgr	Meals	Net Carbs(g)	2 Hrs Bld Sgr	Blood Press	Exercise/Min	Notes/Sickness
Breakfast								
Lunch								
Dinner								
Bedtime								

TUES:	Time	Bld Sgr	Meals	Net Carbs(g)	2 Hrs Bld Sgr	Blood Press	Exercise/Min	Notes/Sickness
Breakfast								
Lunch								
Dinner								
Bedtime								

WED:	Time	Bld Sgr	Meals	Net Carbs(g)	2 Hrs Bld Sgr	Blood Press	Exercise/Min	Notes/Sickness
Breakfast								
Lunch								
Dinner								
Bedtime								

THUR:	Time	Bld Sgr	Meals	Net Carbs(g)	2 Hrs Bld Sgr	Blood Press	Exercise/Min	Notes/Sickness
Breakfast								
Lunch								
Dinner								
Bedtime								

FRI:	Time	Bld Sgr	Meals	Net Carbs(g)	2 Hrs Bld Sgr	Blood Press	Exercise/Min	Notes/Sickness
Breakfast								
Lunch								
Dinner								
Bedtime								

SAT:	Time	Bld Sgr	Meals	Net Carbs(g)	2 Hrs Bld Sgr	Blood Press	Exercise/Min	Notes/Sickness
Breakfast								
Lunch								
Dinner								
Bedtime								

SUN:	Time	Bld Sgr	Meals	Net Carbs(g)	2 Hrs Bld Sgr	Blood Press	Exercise/Min	Notes/Sickness
Breakfast								
Lunch								
Dinner								
Bedtime								

Week 41:
Eye Disease and Diabetes

What Does Science Say about Diabetes and Eye Disease?

Diabetes can affect your eyes and vision; people with diabetes are at much higher risk than the general population for developing *blindness* (retinopathy), *cataracts* (lens cloudiness), and *glaucoma* (pressure inside the eye damaging the optic nerve). *Diabetic retinopathy* develops in people with diabetes, and *hypertensive retinopathy* develops in people with hypertension. Two kinds of diabetic retinopathy have the potential to diminish vision: non-proliferative and proliferative retinopathy. In *non-proliferative retinopathy,* existing blood vessels in the retina deteriorate. Deteriorating blood vessels can become blocked or can develop balloon-like deformities called aneurysms. Fluids, fats, and proteins leak out of the abnormal blood vessels. Fluid can collect in the area of the retina that is responsible for sharp vision (the macula).

Macular swelling (edema) impairs the fine vision necessary for reading and detail work. In *proliferative retinopathy,* new, structurally unstable blood vessels grow on the surface of the retina. These unstable blood vessels cause frequent small hemorrhages (bleeding), causing local irritation with scar formation. In areas that have scarred, the clear mass of gel between the lens and the retina, called the vitreous, can adhere to the retina. These abnormal attachments between the retina and vitreous eventually distort the shape of the vitreous and cause the vitreous to pull against its tethers. This force can pull apart the layers of the retina, so that the retina can't function. This separation of layers is known as retinal detachment and is one of the most serious consequences of proliferative retinopathy. Sudden bleeding into the vitreous also can obscure vision, often quite suddenly.

Why Should I Be Concerned about Eye Disease?

Like *cataracts* and *glaucoma, diabetic retinopathy* takes years to develop, but it is present in close to *80 percent* of people with Type 1 or Type 2 diabetes who are treated with insulin and who have had diabetes for *twenty years or longer.* People who do not require daily insulin to manage blood sugars will be less likely to develop retinopathy, with 20 percent showing eye abnormalities twenty years after they were diagnosed with diabetes. People with diabetic retinopathy usually also have kidney damage caused by diabetes. Diabetic retinopathy is the leading cause of blindness in the United States for people between the ages of twenty and sixty-four.

How Can I Prevent or Minimize Diabetic Eye Disease (Retinopathy)?

Controlling blood sugar and blood pressure are essential to preventing diabetic retinopathy. Doctors monitor blood sugar control by measuring a type of hemoglobin protein in the blood, hemoglobin A1C. If you are able to reduce your blood sugar average by the equivalent of one A1C point, you will reduce your risk for retinopathy by 35 percent over the next ten years. Annual dilated eye exams with an ophthalmologist are crucial for people with diabetes. If either proliferative or non-proliferative retinopathy is discovered during an annual exam, more frequent eye exams are likely to be recommended. Treatment can start before sight is affected and can delay vision impairment.

Diabetes and Eye Disease Information Resources

1. The National Institute of Diabetes and Digestive and Kidney Diseases http://diabetes.niddk.nih.gov/ dm/pubs/complications_eyes/.
2. The National Eye Institute, *Diabetic Retinopathy: What You Should Know,* http://www.nei.nih.gov/ health/diabetic/retinopathy.asp.

Reviewed by: **Jay Krakovitz, M.D.,** for:

DIABETES SELF-DEFENSE, LLC
6360 Quail Street, Denver, CO 80004
Cell: 303-931-9710; **Web:** www.DiabetesSelfDefense.com

Week Beginning: _____

Weekly Record

MON:	Time	Bld Sgr	Meals	Net Carbs(g)	2 Hrs Bld Sgr	Blood Press	Exercise/Min	Notes/Sickness
Breakfast								
Lunch								
Dinner								
Bedtime								

TUES:	Time	Bld Sgr	Meals	Net Carbs(g)	2 Hrs Bld Sgr	Blood Press	Exercise/Min	Notes/Sickness
Breakfast								
Lunch								
Dinner								
Bedtime								

WED:	Time	Bld Sgr	Meals	Net Carbs(g)	2 Hrs Bld Sgr	Blood Press	Exercise/Min	Notes/Sickness
Breakfast								
Lunch								
Dinner								
Bedtime								

THUR:	Time	Bld Sgr	Meals	Net Carbs(g)	2 Hrs Bld Sgr	Blood Press	Exercise/Min	Notes/Sickness
Breakfast								
Lunch								
Dinner								
Bedtime								

FRI:	Time	Bld Sgr	Meals	Net Carbs(g)	2 Hrs Bld Sgr	Blood Press	Exercise/Min	Notes/Sickness
Breakfast								
Lunch								
Dinner								
Bedtime								

SAT:	Time	Bld Sgr	Meals	Net Carbs(g)	2 Hrs Bld Sgr	Blood Press	Exercise/Min	Notes/Sickness
Breakfast								
Lunch								
Dinner								
Bedtime								

SUN:	Time	Bld Sgr	Meals	Net Carbs(g)	2 Hrs Bld Sgr	Blood Press	Exercise/Min	Notes/Sickness
Breakfast								
Lunch								
Dinner								
Bedtime								

Week 42:
Kidney Disease (Nephropathy) and Diabetes

What Does Science Say about Diabetes and Kidney Disease?

Diabetic kidney disease or *nephropathy* is a complication of diabetes. It can occur in people with Type 2 diabetes, the most common diabetes type, or in people with Type 1 diabetes, the type that usually, though not always, begins at an early age and requires insulin. Up to 40 percent of people with Type 1 diabetes eventually develop significant kidney disease, which sometimes requires dialysis or a kidney transplant. A much smaller percentage of people with Type 2 diabetes develop kidney disease. Diabetic kidney disease is caused by damage to the tiniest blood vessels. As kidney disease progresses, proteins leak into the urine, and the kidneys gradually lose their ability to remove waste products from the blood. More than one-third of the fifty thousand people in the United States diagnosed each year with end-stage kidney disease have diabetes.

Why Should I Be Concerned About Kidney Disease?

Kidney disease is a lifelong condition that cannot be reversed once damage is done. The disease is progressive, meaning it continues to get worse. Once kidney disease reaches advanced stages, dialysis or a kidney transplant can become necessary. There are two types of dialysis, a treatment that removes waste products from the blood. *Hemodialysis* usually is done at a dialysis center in three to four hour sessions three times a week. *Peritoneal dialysis* can be done at home. It is a good alternative for some patients, although it requires significant time and self-care.

How Can I Prevent or Minimize Diabetic Kidney Disease?

The best way to prevent diabetic kidney disease is to keep your blood sugar in as close to normal range as possible (80-120 mg/dL). In addition, your blood pressure should be monitored frequently, and high blood pressure (above 130/80) should be treated promptly. Two types of blood pressure medicines protect against kidney damage in ways that go beyond lowering your blood pressure. These medications are excellent choices for controlling blood pressure in people with diabetes. They include angiotensin-converting enzyme inhibitors (ACE inhibitors)—lisinopril (Zestril®, Prinivil®), enalapril (Vasotec®), moexipril (Univasc®), benazepril (Lotensin®) and others—and angiotensin receptor blockers (ARBs), such as losartan (Cozaar®), valsartan (Diovan®) and others.

Avoiding medications that can harm the kidneys like ibuprofen (Advil®, Motrin®) also can help to prevent kidney disease. A low-protein diet (10 percent to 12 percent or less of total calories) also may slow or halt the progression of kidney disease. If you smoke cigarettes, you should quit. Elevated levels of lipids, such as cholesterol, are associated with kidney damage, so you may be able to reduce your risk of diabetic kidney disease by reducing your cholesterol and other lipid levels through diet, exercise, and possibly medication.

Diabetes and Kidney Disease Information Resources

1. The National Institute of Diabetes and Digestive and Kidney Diseases: National Kidney Disease Education Program (www.nkdep.nih.gov)
2. The National Kidney Foundation or www.kidney.org.
3. Aetna Insurance's Consumer Health Information Site, InteliHealth, at http://www.intelihealth.com/IH/ihtIH?t=31110 Andp=~br,IHW|~st,24479|~r,WSIHW000|~b,*|
4. www.kidneycoach.com (A Natural Approach to Managing Kidney Disease)

Reviewed by: **Jay Krakovitz, M.D.,** for:

DIABETES SELF-DEFENSE, LLC
6360 Quail Street, Denver, CO 80004
Cell: 303-931-9710; **Web:** www.DiabetesSelfDefense.com

Week Beginning: _____

Weekly Record

MON:	Time	Bld Sgr	Meals	Net Carbs(g)	2 Hrs Bld Sgr	Blood Press	Exercise/Min	Notes/Sickness
Breakfast								
Lunch								
Dinner								
Bedtime								

TUES:	Time	Bld Sgr	Meals	Net Carbs(g)	2 Hrs Bld Sgr	Blood Press	Exercise/Min	Notes/Sickness
Breakfast								
Lunch								
Dinner								
Bedtime								

WED:	Time	Bld Sgr	Meals	Net Carbs(g)	2 Hrs Bld Sgr	Blood Press	Exercise/Min	Notes/Sickness
Breakfast								
Lunch								
Dinner								
Bedtime								

THUR:	Time	Bld Sgr	Meals	Net Carbs(g)	2 Hrs Bld Sgr	Blood Press	Exercise/Min	Notes/Sickness
Breakfast								
Lunch								
Dinner								
Bedtime								

FRI:	Time	Bld Sgr	Meals	Net Carbs(g)	2 Hrs Bld Sgr	Blood Press	Exercise/Min	Notes/Sickness
Breakfast								
Lunch								
Dinner								
Bedtime								

SAT:	Time	Bld Sgr	Meals	Net Carbs(g)	2 Hrs Bld Sgr	Blood Press	Exercise/Min	Notes/Sickness
Breakfast								
Lunch								
Dinner								
Bedtime								

SUN:	Time	Bld Sgr	Meals	Net Carbs(g)	2 Hrs Bld Sgr	Blood Press	Exercise/Min	Notes/Sickness
Breakfast								
Lunch								
Dinner								
Bedtime								

Week 43:
Nerve Diseases (Neuropathies) and Diabetes

What Does Science Say about Diabetes and Nerve Diseases (Diabetic Neuropathies)?

Diabetic neuropathies include several nerve disorders that affect people with diabetes:

- Peripheral neuropathy—This is the most common type of diabetic neuropathy, affecting the longest (most "peripherally" reaching) nerves in your body. It causes numbness or pain in the feet and lower legs. Symptoms can include numbness, tingling, sharp or burning pain, cramps, hypersensitivity to touch, and problems in balance or coordination.
- Autonomic neuropathy—This neuropathy damages important collections of nerves that control your unconscious body functions. It especially may affect your digestion, your circulation and your sexual function. Symptoms of autonomic neuropathy are varied, depending on which of your automatic body functions have lost their normal nerve control.
- Localized nerve failures (focal neuropathy)—A nerve that controls a single muscle can lose its function. Common symptoms are double vision, drooping of the cheek on one side of the head (commonly known as Bell's palsy), problems with speech and double vision.

Why Should I Worry about Diabetic Neuropathies?

More than half of all people with diabetes have developed some form of neuropathy by the time they have had diabetes for twenty five years. Peripheral and autonomic neuropathies are usually long-term problems, but most cases of focal neuropathy last only a few weeks or months. Diabetic neuropathies occur in both Type 1 and Type 2 diabetes, and they are most common in those whose blood glucose (blood sugar) levels have not been well controlled. Although the various forms of diabetic neuropathy can occur in people who have had diabetes for a short time, they are most likely to affect those who have had the disease for more than a decade, and they are more common in people older than forty. Diabetics who smoke are especially at risk.

How Can I Prevent or Minimize Diabetic Neuropathies?

Because diabetic neuropathy is caused by abnormally high levels of blood glucose, diabetics can help to prevent this problem by tightly controlling their blood sugar. In a ten-year study conducted by the National Institute of Diabetes and Digestive and Kidney Diseases (NIDDK), diabetics who kept their blood glucose levels close to normal (80-120 mg/dL) reduced their risk of peripheral neuropathy by *60 percent*. Avoiding smoking can help to prevent or delay neuropathies, one of several important reasons that people with diabetes should not smoke.

Neuropathies and Diabetes Information Resources

1. The National Institute of Diabetes and Digestive and Kidney Diseases http://diabetes.niddk.nih.gov/dm/pubs/neuropathies/
2. The American Diabetes Association, "Diabetic Neuropathy" at http://www.diabetes.org/living-with-diabetes/complications/neuropathy/

Reviewed by: **Jay Krakovitz, M.D.,** for:

DIABETES SELF-DEFENSE, LLC
6360 Quail Street, Denver, CO 80004
Cell: 303-931-9710; **Web:** www.DiabetesSelfDefense.com

Week Beginning: _____

Weekly Record

MON:	Time	Bld Sgr	Meals	Net Carbs(g)	2 Hrs Bld Sgr	Blood Press	Exercise/Min	Notes/Sickness
Breakfast								
Lunch								
Dinner								
Bedtime								

TUES:	Time	Bld Sgr	Meals	Net Carbs(g)	2 Hrs Bld Sgr	Blood Press	Exercise/Min	Notes/Sickness
Breakfast								
Lunch								
Dinner								
Bedtime								

WED:	Time	Bld Sgr	Meals	Net Carbs(g)	2 Hrs Bld Sgr	Blood Press	Exercise/Min	Notes/Sickness
Breakfast								
Lunch								
Dinner								
Bedtime								

THUR:	Time	Bld Sgr	Meals	Net Carbs(g)	2 Hrs Bld Sgr	Blood Press	Exercise/Min	Notes/Sickness
Breakfast								
Lunch								
Dinner								
Bedtime								

FRI:	Time	Bld Sgr	Meals	Net Carbs(g)	2 Hrs Bld Sgr	Blood Press	Exercise/Min	Notes/Sickness
Breakfast								
Lunch								
Dinner								
Bedtime								

SAT:	Time	Bld Sgr	Meals	Net Carbs(g)	2 Hrs Bld Sgr	Blood Press	Exercise/Min	Notes/Sickness
Breakfast								
Lunch								
Dinner								
Bedtime								

SUN:	Time	Bld Sgr	Meals	Net Carbs(g)	2 Hrs Bld Sgr	Blood Press	Exercise/Min	Notes/Sickness
Breakfast								
Lunch								
Dinner								
Bedtime								

Week 44:
Dental Disease and Diabetes

What Does Science Say about Diabetes and Dental Disease?

People with diabetes are two to three times more likely than non-diabetics to have destructive periodontal disease, such as *periodontitis.* Periodontal disease is a bacterially induced chronic inflammatory disease that destroys connective tissue and bone supporting the teeth and can lead to tooth loss. In fact, a 2002 study published in the *Journal of Periodontology* confirmed recent findings that people with periodontal disease are at a greater risk of systemic diseases such as cardiovascular disease. Researchers found diseased gums released significantly higher levels of bacterial pro-inflammatory components, such as endotoxins, into the bloodstream in patients with severe periodontal disease compared to healthy patients.

As a result, these harmful, bacterial components in the blood could travel to other organs in the body, such as the heart, and cause harm. Signs and symptoms of periodontal disease include bleeding gums; red, swollen, or tender gums; gums that have pulled away from the teeth; pus between the gums when they are compressed; persistent bad breath or bad taste in the mouth; permanent teeth that are loose or moving apart; any change in the way the teeth fit together when the patient bites; and any change in the fit of dentures.

Other diabetes-related conditions affecting the mouth include burning sensations (known as burning mouth syndrome), abnormal wound healing, fungal infections, and dental decay. Of particular concern to dentists and dental hygienists are the effects of diabetes on the health of the gingiva (gums) known as gingivitis.

How Can I Prevent Diabetic Dental Disease?

Because people with diabetes are at greater risk for periodontal disease than the general population, prevention is always the best first step: getting your weight, blood sugar, blood pressure, and cholesterol under control. Secondly, you'll want to be sure you eat a well-balanced diet and maintain good dental hygiene practices, including: flossing and brushing your teeth with a fluoride toothpaste at least twice per day and seeing your dentist at least two times per year for checkups.

What Are the Recommended Treatments for Diabetic Dental Disease?

In the case of periodontal or gum disease, there are several methods of treatment, including deep cleaning of the gums, medications, and surgery. Your regular dentist can refer you to a periodontist, a dentist that specializes in the diagnosis and treatment of periodontal disease.

Diabetes and Dental Disease Information Resources

1. National Institute of Dental and Craniofacial Health, "Diabetes and Oral Health" at http://www.nidcr.nih.gov/OralHealth/Topics/Diabetes/
2. The American Dental Association, "Oral Health Topics," at http://www.ada.org/3069.aspx
3. The American Diabetes Association, "Oral Health and Hygiene," at http://www.diabetes.org/type-2-diabetes/mouth-care.jsp

Reviewed by: **Jay Krakovitz, M.D.,** for:

DIABETES SELF-DEFENSE, LLC
6360 Quail Street, Denver, CO 80004
Cell: 303-931-9710; **Web:** www.DiabetesSelfDefense.com

Week Beginning: _____

Weekly Record

MON:	Time	Bld Sgr	Meals	Net Carbs(g)	2 Hrs Bld Sgr	Blood Press	Exercise/Min	Notes/Sickness
Breakfast								
Lunch								
Dinner								
Bedtime								

TUES:	Time	Bld Sgr	Meals	Net Carbs(g)	2 Hrs Bld Sgr	Blood Press	Exercise/Min	Notes/Sickness
Breakfast								
Lunch								
Dinner								
Bedtime								

WED:	Time	Bld Sgr	Meals	Net Carbs(g)	2 Hrs Bld Sgr	Blood Press	Exercise/Min	Notes/Sickness
Breakfast								
Lunch								
Dinner								
Bedtime								

THUR:	Time	Bld Sgr	Meals	Net Carbs(g)	2 Hrs Bld Sgr	Blood Press	Exercise/Min	Notes/Sickness
Breakfast								
Lunch								
Dinner								
Bedtime								

FRI:	Time	Bld Sgr	Meals	Net Carbs(g)	2 Hrs Bld Sgr	Blood Press	Exercise/Min	Notes/Sickness
Breakfast								
Lunch								
Dinner								
Bedtime								

SAT:	Time	Bld Sgr	Meals	Net Carbs(g)	2 Hrs Bld Sgr	Blood Press	Exercise/Min	Notes/Sickness
Breakfast								
Lunch								
Dinner								
Bedtime								

SUN:	Time	Bld Sgr	Meals	Net Carbs(g)	2 Hrs Bld Sgr	Blood Press	Exercise/Min	Notes/Sickness
Breakfast								
Lunch								
Dinner								
Bedtime								

Week 45:
Foot Care and Diabetes

What Does Science Say about Diabetes and Foot Care?

High blood glucose from diabetes causes two problems that can hurt your feet:

1. *Nerve damage.* One problem is damage to nerves in your legs and feet. With damaged nerves, you might not feel pain, heat, or cold in your legs and feet. A sore or cut on your foot may get worse because you do not know it is there. This lack of feeling is caused by nerve damage, also called diabetic neuropathy. It can lead to a large sore or infection. If left untreated, an infection could progress into gangrene and later require an amputation.
2. *Poor blood flow.* The second problem happens when not enough blood flows to your legs and feet. Poor blood flow makes it hard for a sore or infection to heal. This problem is called peripheral vascular disease. Smoking when you have diabetes makes blood flow problems much worse.

How Should a Person with Diabetes Take Care of Their Feet?

The following represents a checklist for good foot health: (1) *Wash your feet in warm water every day.* Make sure the water is not too hot by testing the temperature with your elbow. Do not soak your feet. Dry your feet well, especially between your toes; (2) *Look at your feet every day to check for cuts, sores, blisters, redness, calluses, or other problems.* Checking every day is even more important if you have nerve damage or poor blood flow. If you cannot bend over or pull your feet up to check them, use a mirror. If you cannot see well, ask someone else to check your feet; (3) *If your skin is dry, rub lotion on your feet after you wash and dry them.* Do not put lotion between your toes; (4) *File corns and calluses gently with an emery board or pumice stone.* Do this after your bath or shower; (5) *Cut your toenails once a week or when needed.* Cut toenails when they are soft from washing. Cut them to the shape of the toe and not too short. File the edges with an emery board; (6) *Always wear shoes or slippers to protect your feet from injuries; (7) Always wear socks or stockings to avoid blisters.* Do not wear socks or knee-high stockings that are too tight below your knee; (8) *Wear shoes that fit well.* Shop for shoes at the end of the day when your feet are bigger. Break in shoes slowly. Wear them one to two hours each day for the first one to two weeks; (9) *Before putting your shoes on, feel the insides to make sure they have no sharp edges or objects that might injure your feet.*

How Can I Prevent Diabetic Foot Problems?

Be sure to: (1) Tell your doctor right away About *any* foot problems; (2) ask your doctor to look at your feet at each diabetes checkup; (3) ask your doctor how your nerve function and circulation are for your legs and feet; (4) ask your doctor to show you the best way to trim your toenails; (5) ask what lotion or cream to use on your legs and feet; (6) if you cannot cut your toenails or you have a foot problem, ask your doctor to send you to a foot doctor. A doctor who cares for feet is called a podiatrist.

Foot Care and Diabetes Information Resources

1. The National Institute of Diabetes and Digestive and Kidney Diseases at http://diabetes.niddk.nih.gov/dm/pubs/complications_feet/index.htm
2. The American Diabetes Association, "Foot Care," at http://www.diabetes.org/living-with-diabetes/complications/foot-complications/foot-care.html

Reviewed by: **Jay Krakovitz, M.D.,** for:

DIABETES SELF-DEFENSE, LLC
6360 Quail Street, Denver, CO 80004
Cell: 303-931-9710; **Web:** www.DiabetesSelfDefense.com

Week Beginning: _____

Weekly Record

MON:	Time	Bld Sgr	Meals	Net Carbs(g)	2 Hrs Bld Sgr	Blood Press	Exercise/Min	Notes/Sickness
Breakfast								
Lunch								
Dinner								
Bedtime								

TUES:	Time	Bld Sgr	Meals	Net Carbs(g)	2 Hrs Bld Sgr	Blood Press	Exercise/Min	Notes/Sickness
Breakfast								
Lunch								
Dinner								
Bedtime								

WED:	Time	Bld Sgr	Meals	Net Carbs(g)	2 Hrs Bld Sgr	Blood Press	Exercise/Min	Notes/Sickness
Breakfast								
Lunch								
Dinner								
Bedtime								

THUR:	Time	Bld Sgr	Meals	Net Carbs(g)	2 Hrs Bld Sgr	Blood Press	Exercise/Min	Notes/Sickness
Breakfast								
Lunch								
Dinner								
Bedtime								

FRI:	Time	Bld Sgr	Meals	Net Carbs(g)	2 Hrs Bld Sgr	Blood Press	Exercise/Min	Notes/Sickness
Breakfast								
Lunch								
Dinner								
Bedtime								

SAT:	Time	Bld Sgr	Meals	Net Carbs(g)	2 Hrs Bld Sgr	Blood Press	Exercise/Min	Notes/Sickness
Breakfast								
Lunch								
Dinner								
Bedtime								

SUN:	Time	Bld Sgr	Meals	Net Carbs(g)	2 Hrs Bld Sgr	Blood Press	Exercise/Min	Notes/Sickness
Breakfast								
Lunch								
Dinner								
Bedtime								

Week 46:
The Immune System and Diabetes

What Does Science Say about Diabetes and the Immune System?

People with diabetes are at increased risk of developing certain types of infections, particularly those of the skin, urinary tract, and respiratory tract (including the lungs). Before insulin and antibiotics were available, infections were a common cause of death in people with diabetes. Even now, with effective diabetes treatments and many types of antibiotics, people with diabetes are more susceptible to infections than people without diabetes.

And people with diabetes do not recover from infections as easily as the non-diabetic population. Tuberculosis, fungi (including those that cause candida and yeast infections) and staphylococcus (which causes abscesses and boils) are known to affect people with diabetes more than the general population. In addition, people with some diabetes complications, particularly decreased blood flow to the feet and limited sensation in the feet, are more susceptible to serious foot infections.

Why Should I Be Concerned about My Immune System?

Although many factors affect the body's ability to fight infections, a number of studies have shown that the body's defenses do not work as well against infection when blood sugar levels are high. For example, the rate at which white blood cells kill bacteria and fungi is directly related to the blood sugar level: the higher the blood sugar gets, the slower the white blood cells work. The best defense against infection for a person with diabetes is keeping blood sugar levels as close to the normal range (80-120 mg/dL) as possible.

High blood sugar levels make people with diabetes more vulnerable to infections. However, a person's resistance to infections is considered normal when his diabetes is under good control and his immunizations are current. A separate but related issue is that blood sugar levels tend to run high during infections; it is important for all people with diabetes to discuss "sick day" treatment with their diabetes healthcare team. It is also important to maintain good hygiene habits for your skin and feet on a daily basis, paying careful attention to any cuts or scrapes, especially on the bottom of your feet.

How Can a Person with Diabetes Strengthen Their Immune System?

In addition to normalizing blood sugar levels to the 80-120 mg/dL range, regular exercise has been shown to clinically strengthen the immune system, and the exercise need not be heavy or intense. From a nutritional perspective, there have been some new published studies that show probiotic foods like yogurt and other dairy products, with live and active bacterial cultures, can help strengthen the immune system, so it could be a good thing to include a low-sugar or light yogurt in your diet on a regular basis and/or take proven probiotic supplements like those developed by Rob Keller, MD; more information on Dr. Keller's supplements can be found on our website, www.DiabetesSelfDefense.com.

The Immune System and Diabetes Information Resources

1. Goldstein, David E., MD, "Diabetes: A Compromised Immune System," Diabetes Self-Management, July/August 1999
2. WebMD, "Probiotics to the Rescue," at http://www.webmd.com/food-recipes/features/bacterial-prescriptions

Week Beginning: _____

Weekly Record

MON:	Time	Bld Sgr	Meals	Net Carbs(g)	2 Hrs Bld Sgr	Blood Press	Exercise/Min	Notes/Sickness
Breakfast								
Lunch								
Dinner								
Bedtime								

TUES:	Time	Bld Sgr	Meals	Net Carbs(g)	2 Hrs Bld Sgr	Blood Press	Exercise/Min	Notes/Sickness
Breakfast								
Lunch								
Dinner								
Bedtime								

WED:	Time	Bld Sgr	Meals	Net Carbs(g)	2 Hrs Bld Sgr	Blood Press	Exercise/Min	Notes/Sickness
Breakfast								
Lunch								
Dinner								
Bedtime								

THUR:	Time	Bld Sgr	Meals	Net Carbs(g)	2 Hrs Bld Sgr	Blood Press	Exercise/Min	Notes/Sickness
Breakfast								
Lunch								
Dinner								
Bedtime								

FRI:	Time	Bld Sgr	Meals	Net Carbs(g)	2 Hrs Bld Sgr	Blood Press	Exercise/Min	Notes/Sickness
Breakfast								
Lunch								
Dinner								
Bedtime								

SAT:	Time	Bld Sgr	Meals	Net Carbs(g)	2 Hrs Bld Sgr	Blood Press	Exercise/Min	Notes/Sickness
Breakfast								
Lunch								
Dinner								
Bedtime								

SUN:	Time	Bld Sgr	Meals	Net Carbs(g)	2 Hrs Bld Sgr	Blood Press	Exercise/Min	Notes/Sickness
Breakfast								
Lunch								
Dinner								
Bedtime								

Week 47:
Cancer and Diabetes

What Does Science Say about Diabetes and Cancer?

There is recent information on people with diabetes having an increased risk from certain forms of cancer, as detailed below. So in addition to having to worry about the many well-known complications of diabetes—such as heart disease, blindness, amputations, and kidney disease—people with diabetes now need to also be aware of increased cancer risk. Fortunately, many of the recommended therapies for diabetes—such as high-fiber, low-fat nutrition, and regular exercise—can also help in fighting the war against cancer.

Why Should I Be Concerned about Cancer if I Have Diabetes?

Diabetes appears to increase the risk of death from a number of types of cancer, new research suggests. Moreover, this holds true even after accounting for obesity, which is common among diabetics and is a well-known risk factor for cancer.

"Several studies have suggested that diabetes mellitus may alter the risk of developing a variety of cancers, and the associations are biologically plausible," Dr. Steven S. Coughlin and colleagues from the Centers for Disease Control and Prevention in Atlanta point out. To investigate further, the researchers examined the relationship between diabetes and death from cancer in a group of 467,922 men and 588,321 women who were cancer-free when the study began in 1982. The findings are published in the *American Journal of Epidemiology*.

After sixteen years of follow-up, the authors uncovered a link between diabetes and death from colon and pancreatic cancers. In addition, in men diabetes seemed to increase the death risk from liver and bladder cancers, whereas in women an association with death from breast cancer was seen. The researchers note that study had a number of limitations, but conclude that the findings "may help to clarify cancer risks for men and women with a history of diabetes mellitus."

Also, a study released by the *Journal of the American Medical Association* in January 2005 revealed that a study of more than 1 million South Koreans suggests diabetes can raise the risk of developing and dying from several types of cancer, including digestive-tract tumors; the highest risks for developing cancer and dying from it were found in people with the highest blood sugar levels, the South Korean researchers found.

How Can I Prevent or Minimize My Chances of Cancer?

As a person with diabetes, *regular medical examinations* are the first step. According to the American Cancer Society and the American Diabetes Association, there is no magic bullet than can guarantee no cancer, but there are certain steps people with diabetes can take to help minimize their risk, which include: (1) stop smoking; (2) avoid overexposure to the sun; (3) keep blood sugars in as close to normal (80-120 mg/dL) as possible;(4) achieve a body mass index of twenty five or less by losing excess weight; (5) eat a low-fat, high-fiber diet rich in fruits and vegetables; (6) exercise daily for twenty minutes or more; and (7) avoid excess alcohol consumption (more than two drinks per day).

Diabetes and Cancer Information Resources

1. Coughlin, Steven S., et al, *American Journal of Epidemiology* 2004; 159:1160-1167, at www.aje.oupjournals.org, search "coughlin diabetes."
2. Jee, Sun Ha, et al, "Fasting Serum Glucose Level and Cancer Risk in Korean Men and Women," *Journal of the American Medical Association* 2005;293:194-202, at http://jama.ama-assn.org/cgi/content/abstract/293/2/194
3. Denoon, Daniel J., "Why Does Diabetes Raise Cancer Risk?" June 16, 2010, at http://www.webmd.com/food-recipes/features/bacterial-prescriptions

<table>
<tr><td colspan="2">Reviewed by: Jay Krakovitz, M.D., for:

DIABETES SELF-DEFENSE, LLC
6360 Quail Street, Denver, CO 80004
Cell: 303-931-9710; Web: www.DiabetesSelfDefense.com</td></tr>
</table>

Week Beginning: _____

Weekly Record

MON:	Time	Bld Sgr	Meals	Net Carbs(g)	2 Hrs Bld Sgr	Blood Press	Exercise/Min	Notes/Sickness
Breakfast								
Lunch								
Dinner								
Bedtime								

TUES:	Time	Bld Sgr	Meals	Net Carbs(g)	2 Hrs Bld Sgr	Blood Press	Exercise/Min	Notes/Sickness
Breakfast								
Lunch								
Dinner								
Bedtime								

WED:	Time	Bld Sgr	Meals	Net Carbs(g)	2 Hrs Bld Sgr	Blood Press	Exercise/Min	Notes/Sickness
Breakfast								
Lunch								
Dinner								
Bedtime								

THUR:	Time	Bld Sgr	Meals	Net Carbs(g)	2 Hrs Bld Sgr	Blood Press	Exercise/Min	Notes/Sickness
Breakfast								
Lunch								
Dinner								
Bedtime								

FRI:	Time	Bld Sgr	Meals	Net Carbs(g)	2 Hrs Bld Sgr	Blood Press	Exercise/Min	Notes/Sickness
Breakfast								
Lunch								
Dinner								
Bedtime								

SAT:	Time	Bld Sgr	Meals	Net Carbs(g)	2 Hrs Bld Sgr	Blood Press	Exercise/Min	Notes/Sickness
Breakfast								
Lunch								
Dinner								
Bedtime								

SUN:	Time	Bld Sgr	Meals	Net Carbs(g)	2 Hrs Bld Sgr	Blood Press	Exercise/Min	Notes/Sickness
Breakfast								
Lunch								
Dinner								
Bedtime								

Week 48:
Children and Diabetes

What Does Science Say about Diabetes and Children?

Type 2 diabetes could become the most widespread, and potentially devastating, disease to attack America's kids since polio. The number of children (and adults) with Type 2 diabetes mellitus has been growing considerably in recent years. This condition used to be known as "adult-onset diabetes" because it was so uncommon among children and adolescents. Since the 1990s, however, more cases of Type 2 diabetes mellitus are being diagnosed in children than ever before.

And it may only get worse. Because of *rising obesity and lack of exercise*, the Centers for Disease Control and Prevention recently predicted that, unless current trends change, at least one in three American children born in the year 2000 will develop diabetes sometime in their lifetime. That's potentially 1.3 million of the 4 million three-year-olds in the US. Among African-American, Hispanic, Asian, and Native American children, the odds are closer to one in two, or every other child, says K. M. Venkat Narayan, chief of the CDC's diabetes epidemiology section.

"The fact that the diabetes epidemic has been raging was well known to us. But looking at the risk in these terms was very shocking," he says.

Why Should I Be Concerned about Diabetes among Children?

Because kids with Type 2 diabetes face adult-size complications. When Canadian researchers followed fifty-one Native Americans, ages eighteen to thirty three, who had developed Type 2 before age seventeen, they found three on dialysis for kidney failure, one who was blind at age twenty six, one who had a toe amputated, two who died of heart attacks, and twenty-one of fifty-six pregnancies that ended in miscarriage or stillbirth.

"Our worst fears are being realized," says David Ludwig, MD, director of the OWL Clinic. "We're getting the first reports of people who were diagnosed as teenagers and who've had diabetes for ten years. They're now in their late twenties and, as feared, they are developing kidney failure, and some have required amputations. And they're dying at a higher-than-expected rate."

Perhaps the gravest and most overlooked danger: Because of high blood-sugar and insulin levels, twenty-year-old diabetics have cardiovascular diseases once found only in older, out-of-shape adults, such as high blood pressure, high cholesterol, and plaque-choked artery walls. This boosts their risk of early heart attacks and stroke.

"It's unprecedented—an impending catastrophe," Ludwig says.

How Can I Help My Children Prevent or Minimize the Onset of Diabetes?

Bottom line: Type 2 diabetes doesn't have to happen to your child. It can be prevented or at least delayed with the same steps proven to keep at-risk adults diabetes-free. All it takes is a family commitment to healthy eating and activity.

"The kids who do best in our obesity treatment program are the ones whose parents are not just supportive but are also participating in the same healthful lifestyle program," Ludwig notes. One reason is that children model adult behavior. If the parent unwinds after work by walking around the block instead of watching TV, for example, the child is more likely to follow suit. "Even if the parents aren't overweight, they can still benefit by decreasing their own risk for diabetes and heart disease through healthful eating and exercise," says Ludwig.

Children and Diabetes Information Resources

1. Children With Diabetes at www.childrenwithdiabetes.com
2. The Juvenile Diabetes Research Foundation www.jdrf.org
3. Prevention.com, "The New Childhood Epidemic—Diabesity," at http://www.prevention.com/health/healthy-living/childhood-diabetes-and-heart-disease

Reviewed by: **Jay Krakovitz, M.D.,** for:

DIABETES SELF-DEFENSE, LLC
6360 Quail Street, Denver, CO 80004
Cell: 303-931-9710; **Web:** www.DiabetesSelfDefense.com

Week Beginning: _____

Weekly Record

MON:	Time	Bld Sgr	Meals	Net Carbs(g)	2 Hrs Bld Sgr	Blood Press	Exercise/Min	Notes/Sickness
Breakfast								
Lunch								
Dinner								
Bedtime								

TUES:	Time	Bld Sgr	Meals	Net Carbs(g)	2 Hrs Bld Sgr	Blood Press	Exercise/Min	Notes/Sickness
Breakfast								
Lunch								
Dinner								
Bedtime								

WED:	Time	Bld Sgr	Meals	Net Carbs(g)	2 Hrs Bld Sgr	Blood Press	Exercise/Min	Notes/Sickness
Breakfast								
Lunch								
Dinner								
Bedtime								

THUR:	Time	Bld Sgr	Meals	Net Carbs(g)	2 Hrs Bld Sgr	Blood Press	Exercise/Min	Notes/Sickness
Breakfast								
Lunch								
Dinner								
Bedtime								

FRI:	Time	Bld Sgr	Meals	Net Carbs(g)	2 Hrs Bld Sgr	Blood Press	Exercise/Min	Notes/Sickness
Breakfast								
Lunch								
Dinner								
Bedtime								

SAT:	Time	Bld Sgr	Meals	Net Carbs(g)	2 Hrs Bld Sgr	Blood Press	Exercise/Min	Notes/Sickness
Breakfast								
Lunch								
Dinner								
Bedtime								

SUN:	Time	Bld Sgr	Meals	Net Carbs(g)	2 Hrs Bld Sgr	Blood Press	Exercise/Min	Notes/Sickness
Breakfast								
Lunch								
Dinner								
Bedtime								

Week 49:
Pregnancy and Diabetes

What Does Science Say about Diabetes During Pregnancy or Gestational Diabetes?

People with diabetes need to take extra care when having a baby. High blood sugar can be harmful to both a mother and her unborn baby. Even *before* you become pregnant, your blood sugar should be close to the normal range. Keeping blood sugar near normal before and during pregnancy helps protect both mother and baby. Your insulin needs may change when you're pregnant.

Your doctor may want you to take more insulin and check your blood sugar more often. If you take diabetes pills, your doctor will switch you to insulin when you're pregnant. As a standard practice during pregnancy, be sure to check your blood sugar both before and two hours after each meal to be sure you are in good control.

If you plan to have a baby:

- Work with your health care team to get your blood sugar as close to the normal range as possible.
- See a doctor who has experience in taking care of pregnant women with diabetes.
- Have your eyes and kidneys checked. Pregnancy can make eye and kidney problems worse.
- Don't smoke, drink alcohol, or use harmful drugs.
- Follow the meal plan you get from your dietitian or diabetes educator to make sure you and your unborn baby have a healthy diet.

If you're already pregnant, see your doctor right away. It's not too late to bring your blood sugar close to normal so that you'll stay healthy during the rest of your pregnancy.

Diabetes and Pregnancy Information Resources

1. The National Diabetes Information Clearinghouse, "What You Need to Know About Gestational Diabetes" or at http://diabetes.niddk.nih.gov/dm/pubs/gestational/
2. The American Diabetes Association, "Diabetes and Pregnancy" or at http://www.diabetes.org/gestational-diabetes/pregancy.jsp

Reviewed by: **Jay Krakovitz, M.D.,** for:

DIABETES SELF-DEFENSE, LLC
6360 Quail Street, Denver, CO 80004
Cell: 303-931-9710; **Web:** www.DiabetesSelfDefense.com

Week Beginning: _____

Weekly Record

MON:	Time	Bld Sgr	Meals	Net Carbs(g)	2 Hrs Bld Sgr	Blood Press	Exercise/Min	Notes/Sickness
Breakfast								
Lunch								
Dinner								
Bedtime								

TUES:	Time	Bld Sgr	Meals	Net Carbs(g)	2 Hrs Bld Sgr	Blood Press	Exercise/Min	Notes/Sickness
Breakfast								
Lunch								
Dinner								
Bedtime								

WED:	Time	Bld Sgr	Meals	Net Carbs(g)	2 Hrs Bld Sgr	Blood Press	Exercise/Min	Notes/Sickness
Breakfast								
Lunch								
Dinner								
Bedtime								

THUR:	Time	Bld Sgr	Meals	Net Carbs(g)	2 Hrs Bld Sgr	Blood Press	Exercise/Min	Notes/Sickness
Breakfast								
Lunch								
Dinner								
Bedtime								

FRI:	Time	Bld Sgr	Meals	Net Carbs(g)	2 Hrs Bld Sgr	Blood Press	Exercise/Min	Notes/Sickness
Breakfast								
Lunch								
Dinner								
Bedtime								

SAT:	Time	Bld Sgr	Meals	Net Carbs(g)	2 Hrs Bld Sgr	Blood Press	Exercise/Min	Notes/Sickness
Breakfast								
Lunch								
Dinner								
Bedtime								

SUN:	Time	Bld Sgr	Meals	Net Carbs(g)	2 Hrs Bld Sgr	Blood Press	Exercise/Min	Notes/Sickness
Breakfast								
Lunch								
Dinner								
Bedtime								

Week 50:
Financial Help for Diabetes

What Are the Facts about Financial Help for People with Diabetes?

Diabetes treatment is expensive. According to the American Diabetes Association, people who have this disease spend an average of *$2,500 a year* on drugs and medical supplies such as test strips, syringes, insulin, lancets, and insulin pumps. It's a good idea to start by looking for an insurance plan that covers as many diabetes-related expenses as possible. A variety of governmental and nongovernmental programs exist to help, depending on whether you qualify, including the following:

Medicare is a government program providing health care services for people who are sixty-five years and older. People who are disabled or have become disabled also can apply for Medicare, and limited coverage is available for people of all ages with kidney failure. To learn if you're eligible, check with your local Social Security office or call the Medicare Hotline listed below. Medicare now includes coverage for sugar monitors, test strips, and lancets. For more information About Medicare benefits, read the online brochure, "Medicare Coverage of Diabetes Supplies And Services" http://www.medicare.gov/Publications/Pubs/pdf/11022.pdf or contact:

> Health Care Financing Administration (HCFA)
> Office of Beneficiary Relations
> 7500 Security Boulevard, C2-26-12
> Baltimore, MD 21244
> Phone: 1-800-MEDICARE or 1-800-633-4227
> Internet: www.medicare.gov

Medicaid: is a state health assistance program for people based on financial need. Your income must be below a certain level to qualify for Medicaid funds. To apply, talk with a social worker or contact your local department of human services. Check the government pages of your phone book or Google "Medicaid."

Health Insurance: because health insurance is meant to cover unexpected future illnesses, diabetes that has already been diagnosed presents a problem. It is considered a "preexisting condition," so finding coverage may be difficult. Many insurance companies have a specific waiting period during which they do not cover diabetes-related expenses for new enrollees, although they will cover other medical expenses that arise during this time. Recent State and Federal laws, however, may help.

Many states now require insurance companies to cover diabetes supplies and education. The Health Insurance Portability Act, passed by Congress in 1996, limits insurance companies from denying coverage because of a preexisting condition. To find out more about these laws, contact your state insurance regulatory office. This office can also help you find an insurance company that offers individual coverage.

Managed Care: Most HMOs keep costs down by limiting the choice of doctors to those who belong to the network, restricting access to specialists, reducing hospital stays, and emphasizing preventive care. In most managed care plans, especially Medicare HMOs, you select a primary care physician who will be responsible for directing your care and referring you to specialists when he or she feels it's necessary. Some plans also cover extra benefits like prescription drugs. For more information on managed care organizations, particularly the quality of care offered to patients, you may want to contact the National Committee for Quality Assurance (NCQA) at www.ncqa.org on the Internet. Medicare also has many publications to help you learn more about managed care. Go to www.medicare.gov on the Internet for more information.

Week Beginning: _____

Weekly Record

MON:	Time	Bld Sgr	Meals	Net Carbs(g)	2 Hrs Bld Sgr	Blood Press	Exercise/Min	Notes/Sickness
Breakfast								
Lunch								
Dinner								
Bedtime								

TUES:	Time	Bld Sgr	Meals	Net Carbs(g)	2 Hrs Bld Sgr	Blood Press	Exercise/Min	Notes/Sickness
Breakfast								
Lunch								
Dinner								
Bedtime								

WED:	Time	Bld Sgr	Meals	Net Carbs(g)	2 Hrs Bld Sgr	Blood Press	Exercise/Min	Notes/Sickness
Breakfast								
Lunch								
Dinner								
Bedtime								

THUR:	Time	Bld Sgr	Meals	Net Carbs(g)	2 Hrs Bld Sgr	Blood Press	Exercise/Min	Notes/Sickness
Breakfast								
Lunch								
Dinner								
Bedtime								

FRI:	Time	Bld Sgr	Meals	Net Carbs(g)	2 Hrs Bld Sgr	Blood Press	Exercise/Min	Notes/Sickness
Breakfast								
Lunch								
Dinner								
Bedtime								

SAT:	Time	Bld Sgr	Meals	Net Carbs(g)	2 Hrs Bld Sgr	Blood Press	Exercise/Min	Notes/Sickness
Breakfast								
Lunch								
Dinner								
Bedtime								

SUN:	Time	Bld Sgr	Meals	Net Carbs(g)	2 Hrs Bld Sgr	Blood Press	Exercise/Min	Notes/Sickness
Breakfast								
Lunch								
Dinner								
Bedtime								

Week 51:
Traveling with Diabetes

What Is Traveling with Diabetes About?

Planning a trip? Whether you're camping or cruising, you can go anywhere and do almost anything. It just takes a little planning ahead to handle your diabetes. How you prepare depends on where you're going and for how long. Two weeks backpacking through Europe takes different planning than a week at the beach. Will you be crossing time zones? What kind of food will you eat and when? Will you be more active or less active than usual? These are the types of questions you need to answer before you go.

Why Should I Be Concerned about Traveling with Diabetes?

Because you have diabetes, you have special needs that a non-diabetic traveler doesn't, most notably high and low blood sugars. Failing to prepare for traveling—whether for business or vacation—can lead to very serious health problems, especially if your travel is international in nature.

How Should I Prepare for Travel?

Here is a list of tips from the American Diabetes Association:

1. Get a letter from your doctor outlining your medical needs and a prescription for insulin and diabetes pills. Keep your prescription in your purse or wallet.
2. The prescription laws may be very different in other countries and even state to state. If you're going out of the country, write for a list of International Diabetes Federation groups. Write to: IDF, 1 Rue Defaeqz, B-1000, Belgium (www.idf.org).
3. You may want to get a list of English-speaking foreign doctors from the International Association for Medical Assistance to Travelers (IAMAT), 1623 Military Road, #279, Niagara Falls, NY 14304 (www.iamat.org). IAMAT can be reached at 716-754-4883.
4. No matter where you go, wear a medical ID bracelet or necklace that shows you have diabetes. You should also carry an *I Have Diabetes* card in your wallet.
5. Make sure your carry-on bag always has your insulin; plenty of syringes; blood and urine testing supplies; all oral medications (extra supply helps); an airtight packet of peanut butter or cheese crackers, along with glucose tablets/candy for low blood sugar.
6. Notify any airline screener that you have diabetes and are carrying your supplies with you; make sure all medications are well labeled and easily identifiable.

Traveling with Diabetes Information Resources

1. The American Diabetes Association, *Frequent Travelers*, at http://diabetes.org/pre-diabetes/travel/when-you-travel.jsp
2. The American Diabetes Association *Air Travel and Diabetes* at http://www.diabetes.org/living-with-diabetes/know-your-rights/discrimination/public-accommodations/air-travel-and-diabetes/

Week Beginning: _____

Weekly Record

MON:	Time	Bld Sgr	Meals	Net Carbs(g)	2 Hrs Bld Sgr	Blood Press	Exercise/Min	Notes/Sickness
Breakfast								
Lunch								
Dinner								
Bedtime								

TUES:	Time	Bld Sgr	Meals	Net Carbs(g)	2 Hrs Bld Sgr	Blood Press	Exercise/Min	Notes/Sickness
Breakfast								
Lunch								
Dinner								
Bedtime								

WED:	Time	Bld Sgr	Meals	Net Carbs(g)	2 Hrs Bld Sgr	Blood Press	Exercise/Min	Notes/Sickness
Breakfast								
Lunch								
Dinner								
Bedtime								

THUR:	Time	Bld Sgr	Meals	Net Carbs(g)	2 Hrs Bld Sgr	Blood Press	Exercise/Min	Notes/Sickness
Breakfast								
Lunch								
Dinner								
Bedtime								

FRI:	Time	Bld Sgr	Meals	Net Carbs(g)	2 Hrs Bld Sgr	Blood Press	Exercise/Min	Notes/Sickness
Breakfast								
Lunch								
Dinner								
Bedtime								

SAT:	Time	Bld Sgr	Meals	Net Carbs(g)	2 Hrs Bld Sgr	Blood Press	Exercise/Min	Notes/Sickness
Breakfast								
Lunch								
Dinner								
Bedtime								

SUN:	Time	Bld Sgr	Meals	Net Carbs(g)	2 Hrs Bld Sgr	Blood Press	Exercise/Min	Notes/Sickness
Breakfast								
Lunch								
Dinner								
Bedtime								

Week 52:
Annual Diabetes Conferences

What Are Annual Diabetes Conferences About?

In general, there are a few annual diabetes conferences of note: (1) The annual *Scientific Sessions of the American Diabetes Association*, where the latest and greatest scientific findings and products are presented through a variety of papers, seminars, and demonstrations; (2) The *Annual International Diabetes Federation (IDF) World Diabetes Congress*, where pretty much the same agenda takes place, within a more international context. Most of the attendees to these conferences are medical researchers, physicians, diabetes educators, pharmaceutical and medical device companies, medical media, and some actual diabetic patients.

Why Should I Be Concerned about Annual Diabetes Conferences?

Because you have diabetes, you will likely be interested in the latest advances in diabetes management science, including the ever-elusive search for a cure. Ever since 1923, when insulin was discovered by Doctors Banting and Best, the search for a cure for diabetes has been on-going. New drugs, new therapies, and new recommendations are always evolving, so staying on top of the findings at these conferences can help you be aware of the latest diabetes developments and discuss them with your doctor and diabetes healthcare team. Granted, medical science tends to move slowly and cautiously—with good reason—but these conferences provide a gateway to the best medical research and products available for the treatment of diabetes.

How Can I Attend One of These Conferences or Review Their Findings?

Virtually anyone can attend either of these conferences, usually on a one-day basis (ADA) if you are not a healthcare professional. Realistically, though, the vast majority of people with diabetes will not be able to actually attend the conferences, but they can contact these organizations at the links below and get all the information needed from the conferences. Once the conferences are over, usually within a six month period, their findings and papers will be posted on their websites, often including webcasts from the conference/presentation itself.

Annual Diabetes Conferences

1. The American Diabetes Association Annual Scientific Sessions at http://www.diabetes.org/for-media/2011/Sci-Sessions-2011-press-briefing-schedule.html
2. IDF World Diabetes Congress, *http://www.idf.org/worlddiabetescongress/*

Reviewed by: **Jay Krakovitz, M.D.,** for:

DIABETES SELF-DEFENSE, LLC
6360 Quail Street, Denver, CO 80004
Cell: 303-931-9710; **Web:** www.DiabetesSelfDefense.com

Week Beginning: _____

Weekly Record

MON:	Time	Bld Sgr	Meals	Net Carbs(g)	2 Hrs Bld Sgr	Blood Press	Exercise/Min	Notes/Sickness
Breakfast								
Lunch								
Dinner								
Bedtime								

TUES:	Time	Bld Sgr	Meals	Net Carbs(g)	2 Hrs Bld Sgr	Blood Press	Exercise/Min	Notes/Sickness
Breakfast								
Lunch								
Dinner								
Bedtime								

WED:	Time	Bld Sgr	Meals	Net Carbs(g)	2 Hrs Bld Sgr	Blood Press	Exercise/Min	Notes/Sickness
Breakfast								
Lunch								
Dinner								
Bedtime								

THUR:	Time	Bld Sgr	Meals	Net Carbs(g)	2 Hrs Bld Sgr	Blood Press	Exercise/Min	Notes/Sickness
Breakfast								
Lunch								
Dinner								
Bedtime								

FRI:	Time	Bld Sgr	Meals	Net Carbs(g)	2 Hrs Bld Sgr	Blood Press	Exercise/Min	Notes/Sickness
Breakfast								
Lunch								
Dinner								
Bedtime								

SAT:	Time	Bld Sgr	Meals	Net Carbs(g)	2 Hrs Bld Sgr	Blood Press	Exercise/Min	Notes/Sickness
Breakfast								
Lunch								
Dinner								
Bedtime								

SUN:	Time	Bld Sgr	Meals	Net Carbs(g)	2 Hrs Bld Sgr	Blood Press	Exercise/Min	Notes/Sickness
Breakfast								
Lunch								
Dinner								
Bedtime								

Week 53:
The Search for a Cure

What Does Science Say about a Future Cure for Diabetes?

Studies are in process regarding finding a cure for diabetes, and the most promising are those involving pancreatic islet cell transplantation and the creation of an artificial pancreas. The pancreas, an organ about the size of a hand, is located behind the lower part of the stomach. It makes insulin and enzymes that help the body digest and use food. Spread all over the pancreas are clusters of cells called the islets of Langerhans. Islets are made up of two types of cells: alpha cells, which make glucagon, a hormone that raises the level of glucose (sugar) in the blood, and beta cells, which make insulin. Insulin is a hormone that helps the body use glucose for energy. If your beta cells do not produce enough insulin, diabetes will develop.

In Type 1 diabetes, the insulin shortage is caused by an autoimmune process in which the body's immune system destroys the beta cells. In an experimental procedure called islet transplantation, islets are taken from a donor pancreas and transferred into another person. Once implanted, the beta cells in these islets begin to make and release insulin. Researchers hope that islet transplantation will help people with Type 1 diabetes live without daily injections of insulin. Scientists have made many advances in islet transplantation in recent years. Since reporting their findings in the June 2000 issue of the *New England Journal of Medicine*, researchers at the University of Alberta in Edmonton, Canada, have continued to use a procedure called the Edmonton protocol to transplant pancreatic islets into people with Type 1 diabetes.

In the past few years, though, gastric bypass surgery and lap banding—two surgical techniques that reconfigure the digestive system, also known as bariatric surgery—have become very popular and have produced many positive results in terms of helping extremely obese and obese diabetics have their diabetes go into full or partial remission. As with any surgery, though, there are pros and cons that need to be considered. The American Diabetes Association, however, still has many unanswered questions, so for the time being they continue to recommend following the ADA's gold standard of diabetes treatment—diet, exercise, and medication as directed by your doctor.

Even more recently, at the Seventy-First Annual American Diabetes Scientific Sessions in June 2011, there were several positive results presented from artificial pancreas studies conducted at Massachusetts General Hospital and the Mayo Clinic. While these devices are still several years away from commercial use, these recent studies show true promise.

Cure For Diabetes Information

For more information on potential cures for diabetes, see:

1. The National Diabetes Information Clearinghouse (NDIC), *Pancreatic Islet Transplantation*, at http://diabetes.niddk.nih.gov/dm/pubs/pancreaticislet/
2. The American Diabetes Association, "*Is Weight Loss Surgery A Cure For Type 2 Diabetes?*," or at http://www.diabetes.org/for-media/2010/is-weight-loss-surgery-a-cure-for-type-2-diabetes.html
3. www.diabetesincontrol.com, "*Artificial Pancreas May Improve Overnight Control of Diabetes in Adults*," at http://www.diabetesincontrol.com/articles/diabetes-news/10803-artificial-pancreas-may-improve-overnight-control-of-diabetes-in-adults

Appendix

My Things to Do Every Day for Good Diabetes Care

 Follow the healthy eating plan that you and your doctor or dietitian have worked out.

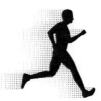 Be active a total of 30 minutes most days. Ask your doctor what activities are best for you.

 Take your medicines as directed.

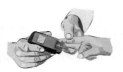 Check your blood glucose every day. Each time you check your blood glucose, write the number in your record book.

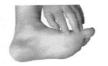 Check your feet every day for cuts, blisters, sores, swelling, redness, or sore toenails.

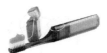 Brush and floss your teeth every day.

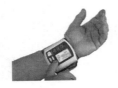 Control your blood pressure and cholesterol.

 Don't smoke.

Source: National Institute of Diabetes and Digestive and Kidney Diseases (NIDDK)

My Medical Exam Checklist—Review with Your Doctor at Each Exam or Check-Up

Your blood glucose records	Show your records to your health care provider. Tell your health care provider if you often have low blood sugar or high blood sugar.
Your weight	Talk with your health care provider about how much you should weigh. Talk about ways to reach your goal that will work for you. Go for common sense goals.
Your blood pressure	The goal for most people with diabetes is less than **130/80** or less. Ask your health care provider about ways to reach your goal, including diet and exercise.
Your diabetes medicines plan	Talk to your health care provider about any problems you have had with your diabetes medicines.
Your feet	Ask your health care provider to check your feet for sores.
Your plan for physical activity	Talk with your health care provider about what you do to stay active.
Your meal plan	Talk about what you eat, how much you eat, and when you eat.
Your feelings	Ask your health care provider about ways to handle stress. If you are feeling sad or unable to cope with problems, ask about how to get help.
Your smoking	If you smoke, talk with your health care provider about how you can quiet.

Source: National Institute of Diabetes and Digestive and Kidney Diseases (NIDDK)

My Annual Medical Exam Checklist—To Be Done One or Two Times Per Year

AIC test	Have this blood test at least twice a year. Your result will tell you what average blood glucose level was for the past 2 to 3 months. The goal is **7.0%** or below.
Blood lipid (fats) lab tests	Get a blood test to check your: • Total cholesterol—aim for **below 200 mg/dL**. • LDL—aim for **below 100 mg/dL; 70 mg/dL** or below is ideal. • HDL—men: aim for **above 40**; women: aim for **above 50** mg/dL. • triglycerides—aim for **below 150** mg/dL.
This test results will help you plan how to prevent heart attack and stroke.	
Kidney function tests	Once a year, get a urine test to check for protein. At least once a year, get a blood test to check for creatinine. The results will tell you how well your kidneys are working.
Dilated eye exam	See an eye care professional once a year for a complete eye exam.
Dental exam	See your dentist twice a year for a cleaning and checkup.
Foot exam	Ask your health care provider to check your feet to make sure your foot nerves and your blood circulation are OK.
Flu shot	Get a flu shot each year as early as possible.
Pneumonia vaccine	Get one, if you're over 64 and your shot was more than 5 years ago, get one more.

Source: National Institute of Diabetes and Digestive and Kidney Diseases (NIDDK)

My Brief Diabetes Profile

Name: _____

Address:_____

Phone: _____ E-Mail: _____

Birthdate: _____

Height: _____

Weight: _____

Type of Diabetes: _____

When/Where First Diagnosed: _____

Doctor Who First Diagnosed Diabetes:_____

Fasting Blood Sugar Level When Diagnosed: _____

Blood Pressure When First Diagnosed: _____

Total Cholesterol When First Diagnosed: _____

Medications Prescribed When First Diagnosed: _____

Current Medications: _____

Last Dilated Eye Exam: _____

Last Dental Check-Up: _____

Last Complete Physical: _____

Minutes of Daily Exercise: _____

Dietary Supplements Taken:_____

Estimated Carbs (grams) Per Meal: _____

Diet Type/Name: _____

Estimated Alcoholic Drinks Per Day: _____

Estimated Hours of Sleep Per Night:_____

Allergies: _____

Last Flu Shot Taken: _____

Last Pneumonia Shot Taken: _____

My Diabetes Health Care Team—Part 1

Medical Professional	Name/Address/Phone/Email
Primary Care Doctor	Name: _____ Address:_____ City/State:_____ Phone: _____ Email: _____
Diabetes Specialist (Endocrinologist)	Name: _____ Address:_____ City/State/Zip: _____ Phone: _____ Email: _____
Ophthalmologist (Eye Doctor, M.D., for annual dilated eye exams)	Name: _____ Address:_____ City/State/Zip: _____ Phone: _____ Email: _____
Certified Diabetes Educator (CDE)	Name: _____ Address:_____ City/State/Zip: _____ Phone: _____ Email: _____
Dentist	Name: _____ Address:_____ City/State/Zip: _____ Phone: _____ Email: _____
Pharmacist	Name: _____ Address:_____ City/State/Zip: _____ Phone: _____ Email: _____
Heart Specialist (Cardiologist)	Name: _____ Address:_____ City/State/Zip: _____ Phone: _____ Email: _____

My Diabetes Health Care Team—Part 2

Medical Professional	Name/Address/Phone/Email
Kidney Doctor (Nephrologist)	Name: _____ Address:_____ City/State:_____ Phone: _____ Email: _____
Foot Doctor (Podiatrist)	Name: _____ Address:_____ City/State/Zip: _____ Phone: _____ Email: _____
Surgeon	Name: _____ Address:_____ City/State/Zip: _____ Phone: _____ Email: _____
Registered Dietitian (R.D., Nutrition Specialist)	Name: _____ Address:_____ City/State/Zip: _____ Phone: _____ Email: _____
Eye Glasses or Contacts Specialist (Optometrist, O.D.)	Name: _____ Address:_____ City/State/Zip: _____ Phone: _____ Email: _____
Alternative Medicine Specialist (N.D.)	Name: _____ Address:_____ City/State/Zip: _____ Phone: _____ Email: _____
Preferred Hospital/Clinic	Name: _____ Address:_____ City/State/Zip: _____ Phone: _____ Email: _____

My Health Care Insurance Information

Insurance Type	Insurance Policy Information
Medical Insurance	Name: _____ Address:_____ City/State/Zip: _____ Cust. Service Phone:_____ Email/Website: _____ Group Name: _____ Group #: _____ Member Name:_____ Member #:_____
Dental Insurance	Name: _____ Address:_____ City/State/Zip: _____ Cust. Service Phone:_____ Email/Website: _____ Group Name: _____ Group #: _____ Member Name:_____ Member #:_____
Vision Care/Vision Plan	Name: _____ Address:_____ City/State/Zip: _____ Cust. Service Phone:_____ Email/Website: _____ Group Name: _____ Group #: _____ Member Name:_____ Member #:_____
Medicare Information **(for USA residents)**	Social Security Number #: _____
Medicare Information **(for USA residents)**	Subscriber #: _____ State: _____

My Medical Exam Records—Page 1

Date					
Purpose					
Primary Care					
Ann'l Physical					
Endocrinlogist					
Weight					
Blood Press					
A1C Bld Sugar					
Cholesterol HDL (good)					
LDL (bad)					
Triglycerides					
Eye Exam					
Dental Exam					
Flu Shot					
Pneu Vaccine					
Other: PSA					
Creatinine					
Microalbumin					
Other:					
Other					
Other:					

My Medical Exam Records—Page 2

Date					
Purpose					
Primary Care					
Ann'l Physical					
Endocrinlogist					
Weight					
Blood Press					
A1C Bld Sugar					
Cholesterol HDL (good)					
LDL (bad)					
Triglycerides					
Eye Exam					
Dental Exam					
Flu Shot					
Pneu Vaccine					
Other: PSA					
Creatinine					
Microalbumin					
Other:					
Other					
Other:					

My Diabetes Medications

Current Medications (RX and Over-the-Counter) and Dietary Supplements

Breakfast	Lunch	Dinner	Bedtime
MEDICATIONS & Dosage			
Example: Humulin R—5 units	Actos—30mg	Humulin R—5 units	Lipitor—20mg
SUPPLEMENTS			
Example—500 IU Fish Oil	1000 IU—Vitamin D	300 mg—Cal/Mag/D	81 mg—baby aspirin

Helpful Diabetes Organizations

1. National Institute of Diabetes and Digestive and Kidney Diseases (NIDDK)

   General inquiries may be addressed to: Office of Communications And Public Liaison
   NIDDK, NIH
   Building 31, Rm 9A06
   31 Center Drive, MSC 2560
   Bethesda, MD 20892-2560
   USA
   For information About NIDDK programs: 301–496–3583 or www.niddk.nih.gov

   The National Institute of Diabetes and Digestive and Kidney Diseases (NIDDK) is the Government's lead agency for diabetes research. The NIDDK operates three information clearinghouses of potential interest to people seeking diabetes information and funds six Diabetes Research and Training Centers and eight Diabetes Endocrinology Research Centers.

2. National Diabetes Information Clearinghouse (NDIC)

   1 Information Way
   Bethesda, MD 20892–3560
   Phone: 1–800–860–8747
   Fax: 703–738–4929
   Email: ndic@info.niddk.nih.gov
   Internet: www.diabetes.niddk.nih.gov

   Mission: To serve as a diabetes information, educational, and referral resource for health professionals and the public. NDIC is a service of the NIDDK. *Materials:* Diabetes education materials are available free or at little cost. Literature searches on myriad subjects related to diabetes are provided. NDIC publishes *Diabetes Dateline*, a quarterly newsletter.

3. The American Diabetes Association (ADA)

   ATTN: Center For Information
   1701 North Beauregard Street
   Alexandria, VA 22311
   Phone: 1-800-DIABETES (1-800-342-2383)
   Web: www.diabetes.org

   Our hours of operation are Monday through Friday, 8:30 a.m–8:00 p.m Eastern Standard Time. The American Diabetes Association is the nation's leading 501(c)3 nonprofit health organization providing diabetes research, information and advocacy. Founded in 1940, the American Diabetes Association conducts programs in all 50 states and the District of Columbia, reaching hundreds of communities. *Mission*: The mission of the Association is to prevent and cure diabetes and to improve the lives of all people affected by diabetes.

A Brief Diabetes Glossary

The following are important terms that are common for people with diabetes and are listed here for quick and easy reference.

ACE inhibitors: Angiotensin Converting Enzyme (ACE) inhibitors, a type of blood-pressure lowering medication that helps slow the progression of diabetes-related kidney disease.

ARBs: Angiotensin II Receptor blockers (ARBs): These medicines block the action of a hormone that causes blood vessels to narrow. As a result, blood vessels may relax and open up. This makes it easier for blood to flow through the vessels, which reduces blood pressure. ARBs are often used in people with type 2 diabetes who cannot tolerate ACE inhibitors.

Beta Cells: The cells in the pancreas that make and release insulin into the bloodstream in response to the amount of glucose, or blood sugar, in the blood. Beta cells are also called islet cells because they are located in areas of the pancreas known as Islets of Langerhans—named after the German doctor that discovered them.

Blood Pressure: When your heart pumps, it forces blood through your blood vessels to get the oxygen-rich blood and nutrients to all parts of your body. This force is called blood pressure. Blood pressure is determined by the amount of blood your heart pumps and the amount of resistance to blood flow in your arteries. Systolic pressure, the top number, shows the force of the blood in the vessels when the heart pumps; the bottom number, or diastolic pressure, is the force when the heart is between beats. According to the latest standards of the American Heart Association, normal blood pressure is less than 120/80.

Bolus: An extra dose of insulin given to help metabolize an unexpected rise in blood sugar after eating, a term normally associated with insulin pump usage.

Byetta®: BYETTA is an injectable prescription medicine that may improve blood sugar (glucose) control in adults with type 2 diabetes mellitus, when used with a diet and exercise program. It can also be used with metformin, a sulfonylurea, or a thiazolidinedione and belongs to a drug class known as incretin mimetics.

Carbohydrate: Along with protein and fat, one of three energy-producing nutrients necessary for good health. Starches and sugars are the main types of carbohydrates. Starches, also called complex carbohydrates, are plant-based foods such as cereals, breads, corn, and potatoes. Sugars, or simple carbohydrates, are the kind found naturally in most fruits and dairy products like milk. Table sugar, cakes, and cookies contain sugar also, but in a refined form that has no nutritional value, so they should be consumed only occasionally.

Carbohydrate Counting: This is a diet program whereby a person counts the number of carbohydrates consumed at each meal or snack occasion; the number of carbohydrates or "carbs" allowed in a day is best determined with your healthcare professional, who will take body size, medications, occupation, and activity levels into consideration. One carbohydrate exchange is 15g of carbohydrate (slice of bread or 1/3 cup of rice).

Cadiac CT: Cardiac computed tomography (to-MOG-rah-fee), or cardiac CT, is a painless test that uses an x-ray machine to take clear, detailed pictures of the heart. This common test is used to look for problems in the heart. During a cardiac CT scan, an x-ray machine will move around your body in a circle. The machine will take a picture of each part of your heart. A computer will put the pictures together to make a three-dimensional (3D) picture of the whole heart.

Cholesterol: Cholesterol is a soft, waxy substance found among the lipids (fats) in the bloodstream and in all your body's cells. It's an important part of a healthy body because it's used to form cell membranes, some hormones, and is needed for other functions. But a high level of cholesterol in the blood—known as hypercholesterolemia—is a major risk factor for coronary heart disease, which can lead to a heart attack. Approximately 70 percent of people with diabetes have high cholesterol.

C-Peptide Test: A simple blood test that determines if a patient has type 1 or type 2 diabetes. C-peptide is an insulin-like protein that is released into the bloodstream during the production of insulin. Although it has no known biologic activity, its level in the blood is a useful indicator of insulin secretion by the pancreas. Patients with type 2 diabetes have high-normal or elevated levels whereas people with type 1 diabetes have low or undetectable levels, indicating little insulin production.

C-Reactive Protein (CRP) Test: The body produces c-reactive protein (CRP) during the general process of inflammation. Therefore, CRP is a "marker" for inflammation, meaning its presence indicates an increased state of inflammation in the body. In studies involving large numbers of patients, CRP levels seem to be correlated with levels of heart disease risk.

Diabetic Neuropathies: Diabetic neuropathies are a family of nerve disorders caused by diabetes. People with diabetes can, over time, develop nerve damage throughout the body. Some people with nerve damage have no symptoms. Others may have symptoms such as pain, tingling, or numbness—loss of feeling—in the hands, arms, feet, and legs. Nerve problems can occur in every organ system, including the digestive tract, heart, and sex organs.

Dialysis: A method of removing waste products from the blood when the kidneys can no longer do so. There are two main forms: (1) hemodialysis, in which the blood flows out of the body and is filtered by a machine, and which is normally done several times per week at a dialysis center; and (2) peritoneal dialysis, in which the blood is filtered through the peritoneum, the tissue lining the abdominal cavity, which can be done at home and which is normally done several times per day.

Diabetic Retinopathy: A disease of the small blood vessels (capillaries) in the retina, the light-sensitive tissue along the back of the eye. Over a long period of time, high levels of blood sugar flowing through the capillaries cause a weakening of these tiny vessel walls. If not corrected, diabetic retinopathy can eventually lead to a complete loss of vision. However, frequent eye exams can detect and treat retinopathy at its earliest stages.

Glucagon: A hormone (body chemical) that raises the level of blood sugar in the bloodstream by stimulating the liver to release glycogen (stored sugar). Glucagon is made by the alpha cells in the pancreas and is released into the bloodstream when blood sugar levels become too low. It can also be injected as a treatment for severe low blood sugar reactions in people who are unable to swallow a rapid-acting sugar.

Glucose: "Blood Sugar" or "Blood Glucose" is a simple sugar made by the body from the carbohydrate in food and carried into the bloodstream. Glucose is the major source of energy for the cells of the body; however, insulin must be present in the bloodstream for the glucose to enter the cells, much like a "lock and key" wherein insulin is the key. Glucose comes from one of two sources: (1) your body's liver, which releases stored sugar; and (2) the foods you eat.

Glycemic Index (GI): The glycemic index measures how *fast* a standard amount of available carbohydrate (50g) in a particular food raises blood sugar relative to pure glucose. Foods with higher index values raise blood sugar more rapidly than foods with lower glycemic index values do. 55 or less is low, 56-69 is medium, and over seventy is high.

Glycemic Load (GL): The glycemic load of a food tells how much eating a single serving of a food raises blood sugar, i.e., a half-cup of rice, a hamburger, or a banana. It is a similar concept as the glycemic index, except that it takes real-world serving sizes into account. It is normally considered a more powerful measure of a food's impact on blood sugar than the Glycemic Index. The standard GL scales says that ten or below is low; eleven-nineteen is medium; and twenty or higher is high for any given food.

Hemoglobin A1C: Hemoglobin to which sugar is attached. Hemoglobin is the protein substance in the red blood cells that carries oxygen. Blood sugar attaches to part of the hemoglobin and remains attached for the life of the red blood cell (About four months). An A1C blood test measures how much blood sugar is attached to hemoglobin, and this number gives an idea of the person's average blood sugar number for the past 2-3 months.

Hyperglycemia: Also known as *high blood sugar*, this occurs when medications, food and exercise are out of balance. Hyperglycemia occurs when there is not enough insulin in the bloodstream or the body cannot utilize the insulin that is there due to insulin resistance. Common symptoms include fatigue, frequent urination, and increased thirst. If blood sugar is 240 mg/dL or below, you can often exercise to lower it. However, if it is above 240 mg/dL and ketones are present, which you can test with a ketone strip in the urine, you should not exercise. Talk to your doctor about the best treatment for your unique case.

Hypertension: Also known as *high blood pressure*, this is blood pressure above the normal range of 120/80 mm/Hg. Up to 73 percent of people with diabetes have hypertension, and it is linked with an increased risk of heart disease, stroke, kidney disease, blindness, and other diabetic complications. Hypertension can be safely controlled with a combination of drugs, dietary measures, and/or exercise.

Hypoglycemia: Also known as *low blood sugar*, this dangerous condition occurs when medication, food, and exercise are out of balance. Common symptoms include feeling weak, shaky, nervous, sweaty, confused and hungry. Severe hypoglycemia can lead to seizures, unconsciousness, or even coma. It occurs mostly among insulin-dependent diabetics but not entirely as some oral medications can induce this condition.

Hyperosmolar Nonketotic State (HHNS): This is a serious condition most frequently seen in older persons. HHNS can happen to people with either type 1 or Type 2 diabetes, but it occurs most often in those with Type 2. HHNS is usually brought on by something else, such as an illness or an infection, and while ketone levels are not out of line, blood sugar levels remain high.

Impaired Glucose Tolerance (IGT): Impaired Glucose Tolerance (IGT) is the name given to define blood sugar (glucose) levels that are higher than normal but below the level of a person with diabetes. It is considered a pre-diabetic state.

Insulin: A hormone made by the pancreas that allows blood sugar to enter body cells and be used for energy. Insulin is made by the beta cells in the pancreas and released into the bloodstream when blood sugar levels rise About the normal range (80-110 mg/dL), such as after a meal. People with Type 1 diabetes no longer produce an insulin in their bodies and must take insulin injections for survival; people with Type 2 diabetes usually produce some insulin, but their bodies have developed a type of insulin resistance that does not allow the insulin to be properly utilized. Up to 40 percent of Type 2 diabetics eventually need to use insulin injections.

Insulin Injections: Injections that are necessary when the pancreas is no longer producing enough insulin for the body to properly use blood glucose. The amount and kind needed must be balanced with the person's food intake and activity level. Different types of insulin are absorbed at different rates—such as very rapid acting, rapid acting, intermediate acting, and long acting—and work for varying periods of time.

Insulin Pump: A medical device that delivers a continuous supply of insulin to the body. The insulin flows through a small, flexible tube connected to a needle which is then inserted into the body. Insulin pumps run on batteries and can be carried in a pocket or worn on a belt.

Insulin Resistance Syndrome: Also known as Syndrome X or metabolic syndrome, a condition that is characterized by four simultaneous conditions known as the deadly quartet—abnormal blood glucose; abnormal blood lipids such as low HDL cholesterol, high LDL cholesterol, or high triglycerides; high blood pressure; and obesity. The theory behind it is that these four conditions often occur as a result of the cells in the body becoming resistant to the action of insulin over a long period of time.

Ketoacidosis: Is a medical emergency that can progress rapidly to diabetic coma and death without prompt hospitalization and treatment; it is a condition where the body is unable to metabolize sugar, leaving high levels in the blood over a long period of time, resulting in the body's burning fat for energy and producing high levels of ketones in the blood. While more common in people with Type 1 diabetes, it can also occur in those with Type 2.

Ketones: Ketones are fatty acids that that build up in the blood as a result of fat being broken down as an emergency energy source. They appear in your urine when your body doesn't have enough insulin in the bloodstream and your blood sugar is extremely high. They are a warning sign that your diabetes is out of control or that you are getting sick. You can test for ketones with a strip that is testing with urine.

Kidneys: Your kidneys are two bean-shaped organs, each about the size of your fist. They are located near the middle of your back, just below the rib cage. The kidneys are sophisticated trash collectors. Every day, your kidneys process about 200 quarts of blood to sift out approximately two quarts of waste products and extra water. The waste and extra water become urine, which flows through your bladder through tubes called ureters. For people with diabetes, the combination of high blood sugar and high blood pressure can damage kidney function and allow protein to leak into the urine.

Liver: The liver is a major organ just beneath the stomach, and its role is to produce a wide range of hormones and assist with fat metabolism.

Macrovascular Complications: Problems caused by disease of the large blood vessels and a common problem for people with diabetes. Heart disease, stroke, periperhal vascular disease, and non-healing foot sores are examples of macrovascular complications that can occur in people with diabetes who have had poorly controlled blood sugar over a period of many years.

Microalbuminuria: This is a condition where small amounts of the protein albumin are found in the urine, indicative of a problem with the kidney's filtering systems. A standard urine test can detect microalbuminuria— which should be completed at least once per year for people with diabetes.

Microvascular Complications: Problems caused by disease of the smallest blood vessels. Diabetic eye disease (retinopathy), kidney disease (nephropathy), and nerve disease (neuropathy) are examples of microvascular complications that can occur in people with diabetes that have had poorly controlled blood sugar over a period of years.

Nephropathy: a medical term for kidney damage that can lead to kidney failure.

Oral Diabetes Medications: Six classes of drugs taken orally to help manage Type 2 diabetes: sulfonlyureas like Glucotrol® (glipizide); biguanides like Glucophage® (metformin); alpha-glucosidase inhibitors like Glyset®; thiazolidinediones like Actos®; meglitinides like Prandin®; and DPP-4 inhibitors, like Januvia®.

Oral Glucose Tolerance Test (OGTT): A medical test in which a person fasts overnight and then drinks a solution containing seventy-five grams of glucose. A diabetes diagnosis is made if two hours later the blood glucose level is 200 mg/dL or more.

Pancreas: An organ, located behind and beneath the lower part of the stomach, that has many important functions, including production of insulin, digestive enzymes, and glucagon.

Pancreatic Islets: Islands of cells in the pancreas that contain insulin-producing beta cells.

Peripheral Neuropathy: A medical term for the slow, progressive loss of sensory nerves in the limbs that cause numbness, tingling, and pain in the hands and legs.

Peripheral Vascular Disease: The medical term for a buildup of fatty deposits and fibrous tissue, called plaques, in the arteries leading to the legs and feet. This can lead to pain in the legs known as intermittent claudication.

Photocoagulation: The medical term for laser treatment of diabetic retinopathy or retinal disease that slows the progression of the eye disease by destroying the new small blood vessels on the retina.

Phytosterols: It sounds almost too good to be true, but we can actually block the cholesterol in foods from entering the bloodstream. Hundreds of research studies document the ability of phytosterols (plant sterols and stanol esters) to safely block the absorption of dietary and liver-produced cholesterol. Plant sterols/

stanols in amounts of two grams per day have been shown to lower both total and LDL ("bad") cholesterol. Phytosterols are available as dietary supplements as well as in foods such as *Take Control®* and *Benecol®* margarines.

Retina: A delicate tissue lining the back of the eye. The retina changes light coming in through the lens of the eye into electrical signals that are sent to the brain where sight is created. It contains many small blood vessels that can be damaged by diabetes.

Type 1 diabetes: A chronic condition in which a person's body makes little or no insulin. Usually an autoimmune disease in which the body's immune system destroys the insulin-producing cells of the pancreas. It usually, but not always, appears before the age of 30. To treat the disease, insulin injections are required. Previous called juvenile diabetes.

Type 2 diabetes: The most common form of diabetes, accounting for 90-95 percent of all cases. It occurs when a person's cells have become resistant to insulin's effects and/or the pancreas does not make enough insulin to meet the body's needs. The majority of those affected are normally older than forty, overweight and sedentary, though not always. Previously known as adult-onset diabetes.